EMBRYOLOGY AND TERATOLOGY OF THE HEART AND THE GREAT ARTERIES

BOERHAAVE SERIES FOR POSTGRADUATE MEDICAL EDUCATION

Vol. 13

PROCEEDINGS OF BOERHAAVE COURSES
ORGANIZED BY
THE FACULTY OF MEDICINE, UNIVERSITY OF LEIDEN,
THE NETHERLANDS

EMBRYOLOGY AND

TERATOLOGY OF THE HEART

AND THE GREAT ARTERIES

CONDUCTING SYSTEM; TRANSPOSITION OF THE GREAT ARTERIES; DUCTUS ARTERIOSUS

EDITED BY

L. H. S. VAN MIEROP, *(Florida)*
A. OPPENHEIMER-DEKKER, *(Leiden)*
C. L. D. CH. BRUINS, *(Leiden)*

LEIDEN UNIVERSITY PRESS
1978

ISBN-13: 978-94-009-9946-6 e-ISBN-13: 978-94-009-9944-2
DOI: 10.1007/978-94-009-9944-2

Cover design: E. Wijnans

Softcover reprint of the hardcover 1st edition 1978

Distributed by Martinus Nijhoff Medical Division, The Hague/Boston/London

PREFACE

The material contained in this book was presented at the Boerhaave Course which was held in Leiden, The Netherlands, on May 2 and 3, 1977. It deals with three topics of considerably recent interest, not only to cardiologists and cardiovascular surgeons, but also to embryologists, anatomists and pathologists.

Papers on the development and the normal anatomy of the conduction system include a discussion of the continuing controversy as to whether discrete and anatomically distinct internodal pathways exist in the human heart. These are followed by descriptions of the abnormal anatomy and relationships of the conduction system in certain complex cardiovascular anomalies. The rather startling discovery that there may be a second, ectopically located and functioning atrioventricular node and common bundle in addition to the usual, but non-functioning one has been of enormous importance in the surgical treatment of certain forms of congenital heart disease.

The panel presentations comprising the first four papers on the topic of transposition of the great arteries highlight the widely differing views and the continuing controversies concerning the nature and pathogenesis of this relatively common and important anomaly. Descriptions of the special morphologic features of ventricular septal defect and pulmonary stenosis as they occur in association with transposition are followed by discussions concerning recent advances in the surgical treatment of transposition, and the common and often troublesome postoperative arrhythmias.

The final section deals with the functional development of the ductus arteriosus and with the pharmacological methods, recently advocated, which attempt either to close the ductus when it remains patent after birth, or to maintain its patency in infants who have a 'ductus dependent' congenital cardiac lesion. Evidence is presented that the use of prostaglandins and possibly also indomethacin may be responsible, indirectly or directly, for structural damage to the ductus wall. These, and other complications, clearly indicate that the drugs are potentially dangerous. They clearly should only be used with a great deal of circumspection in carefully selected cases.

Each of the contributors to this monograph, we believe, is an expert in his field and to each we owe a debt of gratitude for giving so much of their time, effort, and expertise.

Finally our gratitude goes to the Boerhaave Committee for postgraduate education for supplying the stimulus and wherewithal which made the course possible.

L. H. S. VAN MIEROP
A. OPPENHEIMER-DEKKER
C. L. D. CH. BRUINS

CONTENTS

C. Clinical aspects

CONTRIBUTORS

R. H. ANDERSON, Cardiothoracic Institute, Department of Pediatrics, Brompton Hospital, London, United Kingdom.

A. E. BECKER, Department of Pathology, Wilhelmina Gasthuis, University of Amsterdam, Amsterdam, The Netherlands.

W. BERSCH, Institute for Applied Pathology, Speyer, West-Germany.

A. G. BROM, Department of Thoracic Surgery, University Hospital, Leiden, The Netherlands.

C. L. D. CH. BRUINS, Department of Pediatric Cardiology, University Hospital, Leiden, The Netherlands.

F. A. W. VAN GILS, Institute for Embryology and Anatomy, State University, Leiden, The Netherlands.

A. C. GITTENBERGER-DE GROOT, Institute for Embryology and Anatomy, State University, Leiden, The Netherlands.

E. HARINCK, Department of Pediatric Cardiology, Wilhelmina Children's Hospital, Utrecht, The Netherlands.

J. M. J. DE LEERSNIJDER, Department of Thoracic Surgery, University Hospital, Leiden, The Netherlands.

T. G. LOSEKOOT, Department of Pediatric Cardiology, Binnengasthuis, University Hospital, Amsterdam, The Netherlands.

A. J. MOULAERT, Department of Pediatric Cardiology, Wilhelmina Children's Hospital, Utrecht, The Netherlands.

A. OPPENHEIMER-DEKKER, Institute for Embryology and Anatomy, State University, Leiden, The Netherlands.

G. THIENE, Department of Pathology, Medical School, University of Padua, Padua, Italy.

M. J. TYNAN, Department of Pediatric Cardiology, Guy's Hospital, London, United Kingdom.

L. H. S. VAN MIEROP, Department of Pediatrics (Cardiology), University of Florida, College of Medicine, Gainesville, Florida, U.S.A.

A. C. G. WENINK, Institute for Embryology and Anatomy, State University, Leiden, The Netherlands.

J. L. WILKINSON, Department of Child Health, University of Liverpool, Liverpool, United Kingdom.

PART I

CONDUCTING SYSTEM

A. Normal embryology and anatomy

1. EMBRYOLOGY OF THE CONDUCTING SYSTEM

A. C. G. WENINK

INTRODUCTION

Understanding of the development of the cardiac conducting system must of necessity be based upon knowledge of general cardiac embryology. This statement may seem self evident, but in several accounts of cardiac embryology the specialized tissues have been treated as an isolated topic (1, 2). Many authors (3, 4, 5) have dealt with the problem of the earliest possible recognition of the conducting system in embryonic hearts. Unfortunately, the histology of the embryonic specialized tissues is such that it is not easily distinguished from surrounding working myocardium. As a consequence, unequivocal recognition of conducting tissues has been possible only in relatively advanced developmental stages when the definitive form of the heart has been established. Without minimizing the importance of the studies mentioned, it should be noted that they have not attempted to explain important and unusual malformations of the conducting system reported from time to time (6-12). It is perhaps not surprising that descriptions of the conducting system in what could be called nearly final embryonic stages, do not provide an explanation for malformations the development of which must have commenced before these stages were reached.

The developmental concept presently propounded provides an explanation for both the normal heart and congenital malformations (13-16). This is felt to result from following general cardiac development from its earliest stages. In addition, observations on the specialized tissues in other mammals (17, 18, 19) were taken into account.

GENERAL CARDIAC EMBRYOLOGY

For the purpose of this paper, only a schematized account of cardiac development is needed. The most important developmental feature is the evolution of two parallel systems from several primitive cardiac compartments which are serially connected to each other. In downstream sequence, the segments constituting the straight heart tube (Streeter's Horizon X, human embryo of 2 mm CR length, 3 weeks of age) are sinus venosus, atrium, ventricle, bulbus and truncus (fig. 1). The segments can be recognized throughout cardiac development. Thus, a segmental approach to the embryology might be more or less independent of other events like looping, migration and septation. Such an approach will prove to be beneficial for the understanding of congenital malformations.

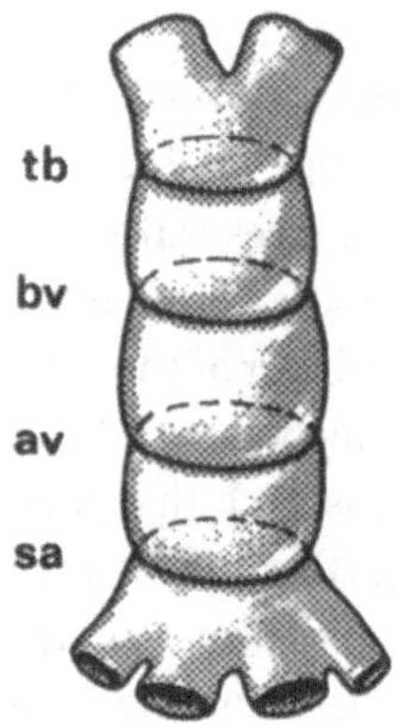

Figure 1. Semischematic representation of the straight heart tube. sa: sinuatrial transition; av: atrioventricular transition; bv: bulboventricular transition; tb: truncobulbar transition.

As will be described below, the primitive anlagen of the conducting tissues are thought to be present as early as the straight heart tube stage. This is the basis for the understanding of the malformations of the conducting system described elsewhere in this book. The question will no longer be where the conducting tissues develop in congenital cardiac malformations, but rather what happens to their primordia during development of such malformations.

Thus regarded, cardiac looping, migration and septation are reduced to more or less secondary events, which determine not only the gross form of the heart (normal or abnormal) but at the same time the disposition of the conducting tissues. The transitional zones between one segment and another are considered good points of reference for the understanding of these developmental events. Looping of the heart tube produces an outer, greater curvature and an inner, lesser curvature. At the outer curvature, the transitional zones are growing apart, whereas in the inner curve they become and remain closer to each other. Thus, the bulboventricular groove becomes very close to the atrioventricular groove in the inner curve. Relative shift of bulbus and atrioventricular canal brings the latter posterior to the bulbus (achieved at approximately Streeter's Horizon XVI, 9 mm, 4½ wks) and a common groove, the so called bulbo-atrioventricular groove is established. The truncobulbar transition (at the level of the future arterial orifices), is also close to this groove. At this very site, disappearance of the myocardium (bulboventricular fold) will normally effect fibrous continuity between an atrioventricular valve and the valve of the posterior artery.

Finally, the septational processes are intended to correspond closely to each other. Thus, posterior and anterior indentations in the atrioventricular canal bring about left and right atrioventricular orifices. Normally, the ventricular septum will correspond to the atrioventricular septum (the ancient septum intermedium of His (20)).

Septation of the bulbus, too, must correspond to ventricular septation, albeit only anteriorly. For, the most proximal portions of the left and right bulbar ridges (which by fusion will form the bulbar septum) are more closely related to the bulboventricular transition than to the ventricular septum (21).

Trabecula septomarginalis and ventricular septum form one structure anteriorly, while diverging posteriorly. Thus, the normal adult heart exhibits a right ventricle of which only the inflow portion is of ventricular origin. The bulbus has formed its outflow portion. The trabecula septomarginalis, which separates the two, is in an entirely different plane from the ventricular septum.

THE EMBRYONIC SPECIALIZED MYOCARDIUM

So far, the intersegmental transitional zones have been described as major points of reference in general cardiac embryology. Now, it will be shown that they are the very sites of origin of the adult conducting tissues. The search for specialized myocardium in embryonic hearts has not been restricted to sites where conducting tissue is known to be present in the normal human adult, but the entirety of the developing heart was screened. Although the earliest specimen in this material was a human embryo of 6.5 mm crown-rump length, it was possible to extrapolate that all four transitional zones between the different compartments of the primary heart tube consist of myocardium with specialized characteristics, i.e. smooth and bright looking cytoplasm with relatively large nuclei showing only slight chromatin staining. The relatively isolated position of the tissue was an additional characteristic.

These four specialized myocardial rings are intersegmental and are therefore termed the sinuatrial, atrioventricular, bulboventricular and truncobulbar rings (Fig. 1).

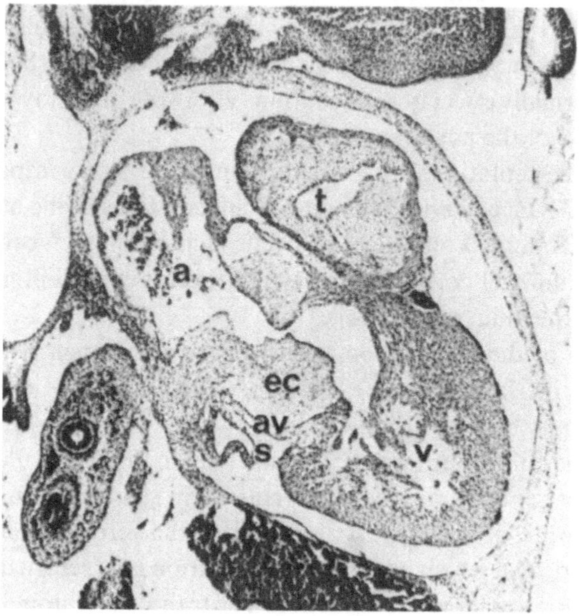

Figure 2. Sagittal section of the heart of a human embryo of 9 mm CR-length, to show the close relationships of the atrioventricular ring tissue (av) with sulcus tissue (s) and endocardial cushion tissue (ec). a: atrium; v: ventricle; t: truncus.

The transitional zones were further characterized by their conspicuous coverings. On their inner side they were marked by endocardial swellings, whereas in the corresponding grooves outside the heart tube accumulations of loose mesenchymal tissue could be distinguished. These intimate relationships with subendocardial tissue on the one hand and the outer sulcus tissue on the other hand remained throughout subsequent development (fig. 2). They are of paramount importance in understanding the adult position of the conducting tissues relative to the fibrous heart skeleton (22, 23, 24).

Here, however, only further development of the specialized rings will briefly be described. Looping of the primitive heart tube and subsequent

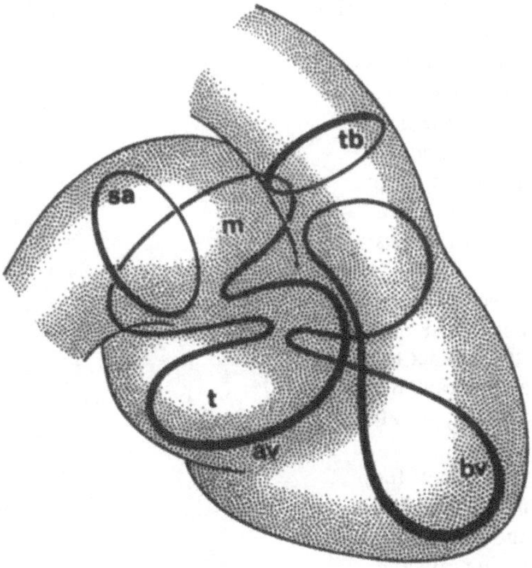

Figure 3. Schematic right lateral view of a normal heart, to show the specialized rings occupying their final positions. sa: sinuatrial ring; av: atrioventricular ring; bv: bulboventricular ring; tb: truncobulbar ring; m: mitral orifice; t: tricuspid orifice.

torsion, migration and septation processes lead to the disposition illustrated in fig. 3. Septation of the atrioventricular canal has effected two indentations in the atrioventricular ring, one anterior, the other posterior. These indentations, which contact each other at the site of the future atrioventricular node, separate the mitral and tricuspid rings.

Invagination of part of the sinus venosus into the right portion of the atrium, brings the sinuatrial ring in contact with the atrioventricular ring musculature. The sinuatrial ring persists as the tissues of the venous valves. Its superior portion gives rise to the sinuatrial node. Its inferior portion, at the site where anterior and posterior indentations of the atrioventricular ring contact each other, produces one of the components of the atrioventricular node (fig. 4).

Looping of the heart tube has produced approximation of the venous and arterial poles. This enables the bulboventricular ring to contact the atrioventricular ring at the right side of the latter. Further migration produces a shift of this contact to the right and, finally, it will be situated at the anterior side of the tricuspid orifice. It will be obvious, that this contact is situated in the bulboventricular fold (fig. 5a and b).

A second contact between these rings is produced by the inferior loop of the

Figure 4. Transverse section of the heart of a human embryo of 16 mm CR-length, to show the components of the atrioventricular node. sa: sinuatrial ring tissue from the right venous valve (arrow); a: anterior indentation of atrioventricular ring; p: posterior indentation of atrioventricular ring; ra: right atrium; vs: ventricular septum.

Figure 5a. Transverse section of the heart of a human embryo of 8 mm CR-length, to show the contact between atrioventricular ring (av) and bulboventricular ring (bv). a: atrium; b: bulbus.

Figure 5b. Transverse section of the heart of a human embryo of 17 mm CR-length, to show the contact between atrioventricular ring (av) and bulboventricular ring (bv). ra: right atrium; vs: ventricular septum.

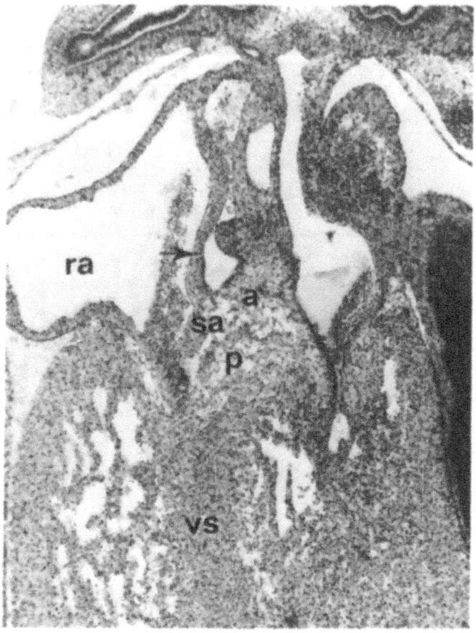

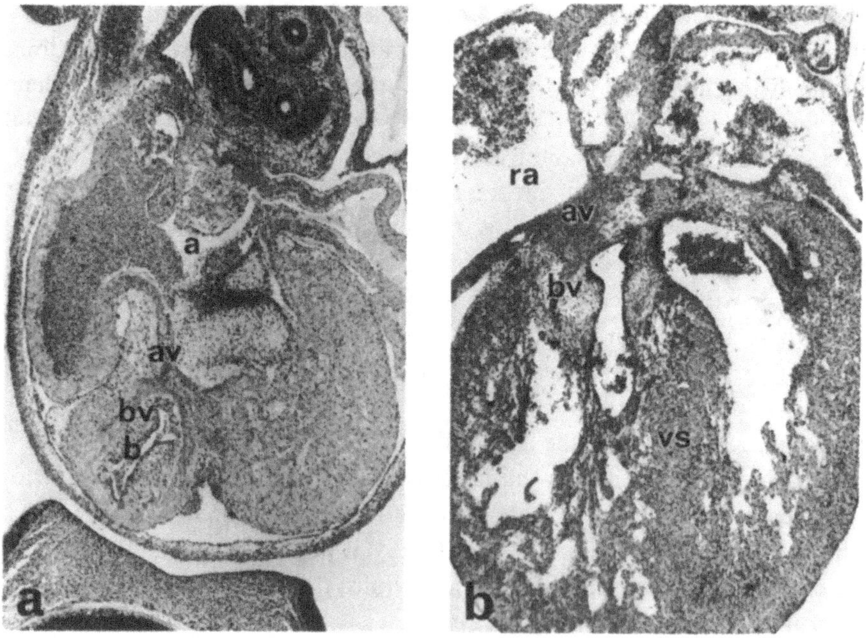

bulboventricular ring, which separates the inflow and outflow portions of the right ventricle. Anteriorly, i.e. where it is covered by the proximal portion of the left bulbar ridge, it is contacted by the developing ventricular septum, and is invaginated posteriorly. On the crest of the septum, this invagination contacts the posterior indentation of the atrioventricular ring (fig. 6).

Finally, in the lesser curvature of the heart loop, the superior portion of the bulboventricular ring is close to the truncobulbar ring. Both rings are in close proximity to the anterior atrial wall.

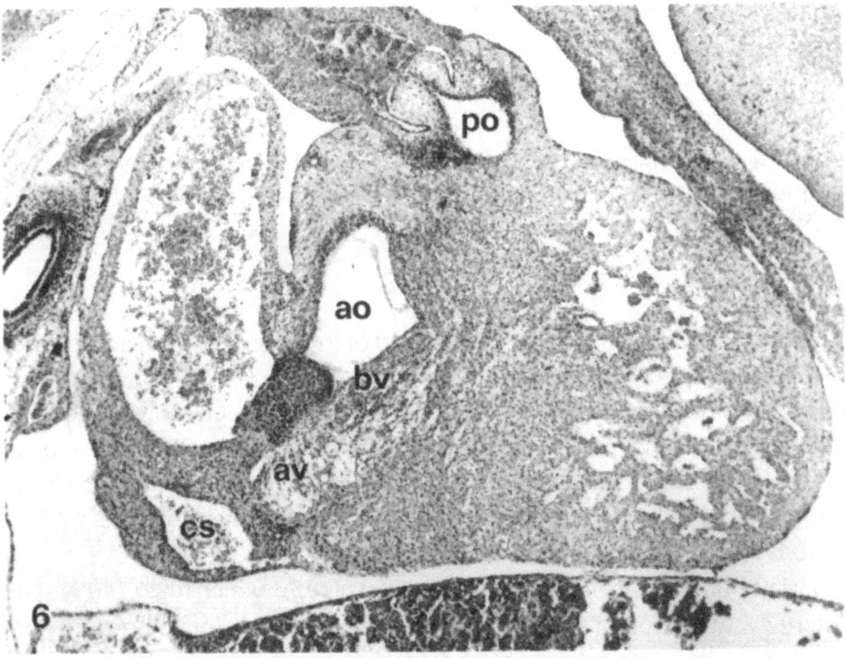

Figure 6. Sagittal section of the heart of a human embryo of 17 mm CR-length, to show the contact between atrioventricular (av) and bulboventricular (bv) rings on top of the ventricular septum (vs). cs: coronary sinus; po: pulmonary orifice; ao: aortic vestibulum.

REMNANTS OF THE SPECIALIZED RINGS IN THE NORMAL ADULT HEART

Only parts of these rings remain preserved in the fully developed normal heart (fig. 7). The sinus node is derived from the superior portion of the sinuatrial

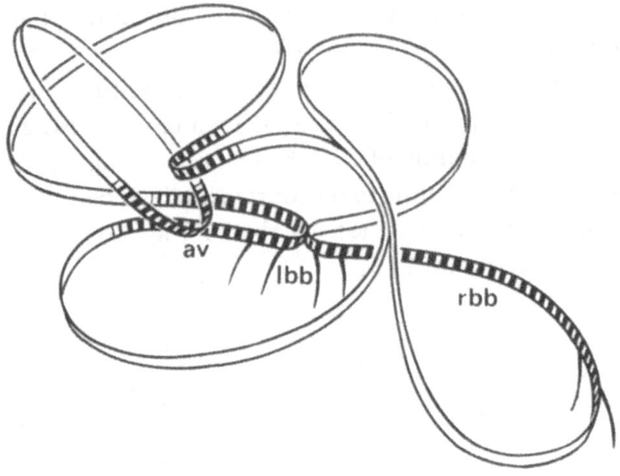

Figure 7. Diagram to visualize the normal fate of the specialized rings. The crosshatched portions form part of the normal conducting system. av: atrioventricular node; rbb: right bundle branch; lbb: left bundle branch.

ring. The atrioventricular node is composed of its inferior portion as well as of both indentations of the atrioventricular ring. The common bundle has its origin in the fused parts of atrioventricular and bulboventricular rings lying on the posterior septum. The right bundle branch is the remnant of the apical portion of bulboventricular ring musculature, and runs through the trabecula septomarginalis. As such, it marks the boundary between inflow and outflow portions of the right ventricle.

The left bundle branch is a relatively new structure, which tails off from the posterior indentation of the atrioventricular ring and the neighbouring portion of the bulboventricular ring. Its development is believed to be an accompanying feature of the ventricular septation. The truncobulbar ring and the superior portion of the bulboventricular ring are not thought to contribute to the normal conducting system.

Finally, it must be stated that the present concept is not as new as it would perhaps seem. Parts of the ring system have previously been described in the developing heart (25, 26). As early as 1923, Benninghoff (27) described these specialized myocardial rings in the hearts of lower vertebrates. He suggested that they were the precursors of the conducting system in mammals. Consequently, the present concept brings together many aspects of cardiac embryology and phylogeny. It is felt to be of great interest that the ventricular septum, which is a relatively new structure in a phylogenetic sense (27) as well as in human embryology, does not primarily contain any specialized myocardium of its own.

DEVELOPMENT OF SPECIALIZED MYOCARDIUM IN CONGENITAL MALFORMATIONS

Elsewhere in this book, the conducting tissues are described in congenital heart block, univentricular hearts, corrected transposition and atrioventricular canal malformations.

The close relationship of specialized myocardium and sulcus tissue is of major importance for the development of congenital block. At two sites the presence of sulcus tissue may cause discontinuities in the conducting tissues. During development of the atrioventricular node, the anterior and posterior indentations of the atrioventricular ring are approximated, but at the same time sulcus tissue is invaginated. This may prevent contact in this region and fibrous tissue may cover the central portion of the node, depriving it of its atrial input. On top of the ventricular septum, the posterior atrioventricular indentation has to contact bulboventricular specialized tissue. Here, too, invagination of sulcus tissue may prevent continuity. This results in an interruption in the penetrating bundle.

Obviously, the continuity of node and bundle on top of the ventricular septum also depends on normal septation of the ventricle. Particularly in univentricular hearts, this septation is grossly disturbed. In some malformations, the bulboventricular transition (the trabecula septomarginalis of the normal heart) is abnormally accentuated. These are the cases with an accessory outlet chamber. In the absence of such an accentuation ('common ventricle'), conducting tissue merely descends along the posterior ventricular wall, like the left bundle branch does along the ventricular septum in normal hearts.

In the presence of an outlet chamber, however, another route of conduction is used. Here the contact between atrioventricular and bulboventricular tissues, anterior to the rightsided atrioventricular orifice, gives rise to an anterior node, from which a bundle continues on the rim of the muscular septum between main and outlet chambers. There is a marked difference between cases with d-loop and those with l-loop, i.e. cases with rightsided outlet chamber and those with left sided outlet chamber (28).

When the outlet chamber is to the right, the apical loop of the bulboventricular ring is used to form the bundle (note that impulse conduction is the reverse of normal). Anterior node and the proximal part of the bundle are well lateral and have no relation with the arterial orifices (fig. 8).

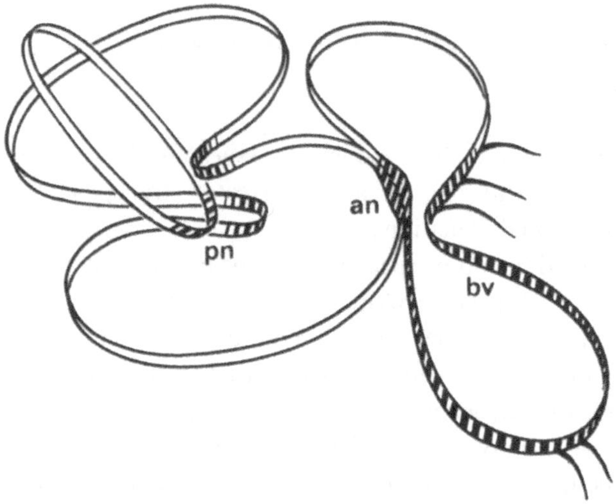

Figure 8. Diagram to visualize the fate of the specialized rings in primitive ventricle with right-sided outlet chamber. The crosshatched portions form the definitive conducting system. pn: posterior node; an: anterior node. Note that invagination of the bulboventricular ring (bv) has been deficient.

In cases with a leftsided outlet chamber, the basal portion of the bulboventricular ring forms the penetrating bundle. This was the portion that was localized in the bulboventricular fold. Now, therefore, there is an intimate relationship of the bundle with the arterial pole. It is situated in the fibrous annulus of the posterior artery, at the site of semilunar-atrioventricular fibrous continuity (fig. 9).

Consequently, there are marked differences according to the site of the outlet chamber. However, it is not always too simple to determine whether an outlet chamber should be considered as right or left, that is whether there is a normal or an inverted bulboventricular loop. This problem probably relates to that of criss-cross atrioventricular relationships (29). In these cases, careful intraoperative mapping is advisable for the surgeon.

Much similarity to primitive ventricle with leftsided outlet chamber is shown by corrected transposition. Here, too, an l-loop is present.

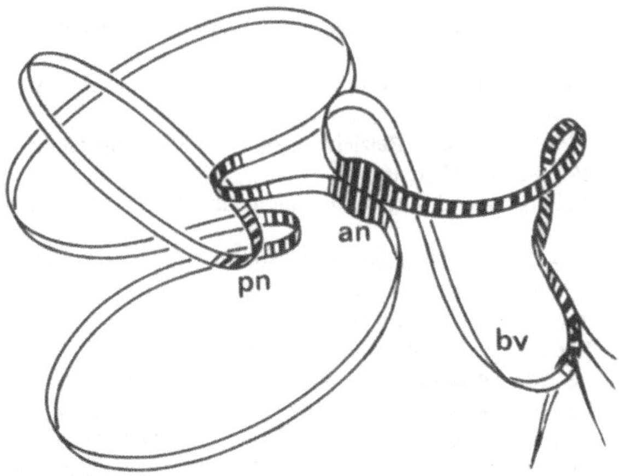

Figure 9. Diagram to visualize the fate of the specialized rings in primitive ventricle with left-sided outlet chamber. The crosshatched portions form the definitive conducting system. pn: posterior node; an: anterior node. Note that the bulboventricular ring (bv) is in an inverted position compared to fig. 8.

Development of a normal penetrating bundle is prevented by malalignment of atrial and ventricular septa.

Instead, the basal portion of the bulboventricular ring (which was situated in the bulboventricular fold) develops into the penetrating bundle. Again, the bundle will pass through the site of semilunar-atrioventricular fibrous continuity and be intimately related to the posterior artery. The occurrence of congenital block in these cases may be explained by the bundle lying at a site, where, normally, only fibrous tissue remains.

Finally, with regard to the conducting tissues in atrioventricular canal malformations, the embryologic considerations will be contained within the chapter on that topic.

REFERENCES

1. Patten, B. M., The development of the heart. In: S. E. Gould (ed.) *Pathology of the heart and blood vessels*. Springfield, Illinois 1968.
2. Los, J. A., Embryology. In: H. Watson (ed.) *Pediatric Cardiology*. London 1968.
3. Mall, F. P., On the development of the heart. *Am. J. Anat.* 94, 73 (1912).
4. Sanabria, T., Recherches sur la différenciation du tissue nodal et connecteur du coeur des mammifères. *Arch. Biol.* 47, 1 (1936).

5. Walls, E. W., The development of the specialized tissue of the human heart. *J. Anat.* 81, 93 (1947).
6. Mönckeberg, J. G., Zur Entwicklungsgeschichte des Atrioventrikular-systems. *Verh. Dtsch. Ges. Pathol.* 18, 228 (1913).
7. Uher, V., Zur Pathologie des Reizleitungssystems bei kongenitalen Herzanomalien. *Frankfurter Z. Pathol.* 49, 347 (1936).
8 Hudson, R. E. B., Surgical pathology of the conducting system of the heart. *Br. Heart J.* 29, 646 (1967).
9. Anderson, R. H., Arnold, R., Thapar, M. K., Jones, R. S. and Hamilton, D. I., Cardiac specialized tissue in hearts with an apparently single ventricular chamber (Double inlet left ventricle). *Am. J. Cardiol.* 33, 95 (1974).
10. Anderson, R. H., Becker, A. E., Arnold, R. and Wilkinson, J. L. The conducting tissues in congenitally corrected transposition. *Circulation* 50, 911 (1974).
11. Bharati, S. and Lev, M. The course of the conducting system in single ventricle with inverted (L-)loop and inverted (L-)transposition. *Circulation* 51, 723 (1975).
12. Baissus, C., Latour, H., Puech, P. and Grolleau-Roux, R. Dualité embryologique des voies nodo-hisiennes: son rôle en pathologie. *Arch. Mal. Coeur* 68-9, 953 (1975).
13. Anderson, R. H., Becker, A. E., Wenink, A. C. G. and Janse, M. J. The development of the cardiac specialized tissue. In: Wellens, Lie and Janse (ed.) *The conduction system of the heart. Structure, function and clinical implications*, Leiden 1976.
14. Wenink, A. C. G. Development of the human cardiac conducting system. *J. Anat.* 121, 617 (1976).
15. Wenink, A. C. G. Le développement des voies de conduction atrioventriculaire. *Bull. Assoc. Anat.* 60, 623 (1977).
16. Anderson, R. H., Becker, A. E. and Wenink, A. C. G. The development of the conducting tissues. In: Roberts and Gelband (ed.) *Cardiac arrhythmias in the neonate, infant and child.* New York 1977.
17. Shaner, R. F. The development of the atrioventricular node, bundle of His and sinuatrial node in the calf, with a description of a third, embryonic node-like structure. *Anat. Rec.* 44, 85 (1929).
18. Gossrau, R. Über zusätzliches Reizleitungsgewebe im Goldhamsterherzen. *Z. Zellforsch. Mikrosk. Anat.* 115, 587 (1971).
19. Anderson, R. H. The disposition, morphology and innervation of cardiac specialized tissue in the guinea pig. *J. Anat.* 111, 453 (1972).
20. His, W. *Beiträge zur Anatomie des menschlichen Herzens.* pp. 10-14, Leipzig 1886.
21. Wenink, A. C. G., The medial papillary complex. *Br. Heart J.* 39-9. 1012 (1977).
22. Wenink, A. C. G. *Some details on the final stages of heart septation in the human embryo.* Thesis Leiden 1971.
23. Wenink, A. C. G. La formation du septum membranaceum dans le coeur humain. *Bull. Assoc. Anat.* 58, 1127 (1974).
24. Anderson, R. H., Wenink, A. C. G., Losekoot, T. G. and Becker, A. E. Congenitally complete heart block. Developmental aspects. *Circulation* 56-1, 90 (1977).
25. Keith, A. and Flack, M. The form and nature of the muscular connections between the primary divisions of the vertebrate heart. *J. Anat. Physiol.* 41, 172 (1907).
26. Anderson, R. H. and Taylor, I. M. Development of atrioventricular specialized tissue in the human heart. *Br. Heart J.* 34, 1205 (1972).
27. Benninghoff, A. Über die Beziehungen des Reizleitungssystems und der Papillarmuskeln zu den Konturfasern des Herzschlauches. *Anat. Anz.* 57, Ergänzungsheft 185: 208 (1923).
28. Wenink, A. C. G. The conducting tissues in primitive ventricle with outlet chamber. Two different possibilities. *J. Thorac. Cardiovasc. Surg.* 75, 747 (1978).
29. Anderson, R. H., Shinebourne, E. A. and Gerlis, L. M. Criss-cross atrioventricular relationships producing paradoxical atrioventricular concordance or discordance. Their significance to nomenclature of congenital heart disease. *Circulation* 50, 176 (1974).

2. THE SPECIALIZED MYOCARDIUM IN THE FOETAL HEART

A. C. GITTENBERGER-DE GROOT AND A. C. G. WENINK

INTRODUCTION

The human cardiac conducting system develops from four rings of specialized myocardium (see Wenink, this book, page 3). Looping of the heart tube in the embryonic period leads to a rearrangement of these rings, followed by a gradual process during which part of the embryonic ring tissue disappears. A few data referring to the intermediate stage seen in the foetus are found in the literature (1, 2, 3). A better knowledge of this phase will enable us to obtain more insight into the transformation of the embryonic configuration into the condition encountered in the neonatal and adult heart.

MATERIAL AND METHODS

The material studied consisted of nine hearts from human foetuses, ranging from 95 to 230 mm crown-rump length (table 1). In some hearts the lateral part had been removed prior to sectioning, leaving only the septal part and the great ostia to be studied. All material had been fixed in alcohol/glycerine and was embedded in parafin or paraplast before making serial sections (10 μm).

In some of the microseries alternate sections were stained with haematoxylin-eosin; Azan; Van Gieson elastic tissue stain; and a modified elastic tissue stain (4) consisting of resorcin-fuchsin, ironhaematoxylin, picric-acid and thiazin-red, while in others only the last staining technique was performed.

To provide better insight into the distribution of the specialized myocardial tissue in these foetal hearts, a graphic reconstruction was made of one case, showing the specialized tracts in relation to the surrounding structures.

Table 1. Material

no	*micro-serie*	*C-R length mm*	*part. sectioned*	*staining techn.*	*BB and MUS*	*L-AVR*	*R-AVR*	*remarks*
1	2360	230	part VS + AS + art. ost.	HE, RF Azan RF etc.	L	—	±	lateral parts heart missing
2	2361	210	part VS + AS + art. ost.	RF etc.	C	—	±	lateral parts heart missing
3	2373	190	heart + mediastinum	RF etc	R	±	+	lacerated
4	2372	170	heart + mediastinum	RF etc.	L	+	+	tracts pale cells in AS
5	2364	125	heart + mediastinum	RF etc.	L	±	+	tracts pale cells in AS (reconstruction fig. 3)
6	2363	115	heart + mediastinum	RF etc.	L	—	+	
7	2501	110	heart-lung specimen	HE, RF Azan RF etc.	L	±	+	
8	2374	105	heart + mediastinum	Azan, RF RF etc.	L	±	+	
9	2362	95	heart + mediastinum	RF etc.	L	±	+	

BB = branching bundle; MUS = muscular ventricular septum; L = left; C = central; R = right; L-AVR = left atrioventricular ring; R-AVR = right atrioventricular ring; VS = ventricular septum; AS = atrial septum; HE = haematoxylin and eosin; RF = resorcin-fuchsin; RF etc. = resorcin-fuchsin, ironhaematoxylin, picric acid and thiazin-red.

OBSERVATIONS

All features of the conducting system in the adult heart were present in the foetal hearts studied. The adult condition is characterized by a sinuatrial node and an atrioventricular junctional area comprising a transitional cell zone, a compound node, a penetrating bundle and a branching bundle giving rise to a right and left bundle branch (5, 6). In the foetal hearts, however, some additional specialized myocardial tissue was encountered.

The configuration of the specialized myocardium in the nine foetal hearts will be described in general, from ventricular to atrial level. Table 1 provides information on each separate foetus.

The right and left bundle branch, surrounded by scanty to fairly abundant connective tissue, converge to form the branching bundle. In histology and distribution both resemble the infant condition. There proved to be a varying relationship between the branching bundle, and with it the right and left bundle branch, and the muscular ventricular septum. In seven cases the branching bundle was situated more to the left on the septum, as at the right

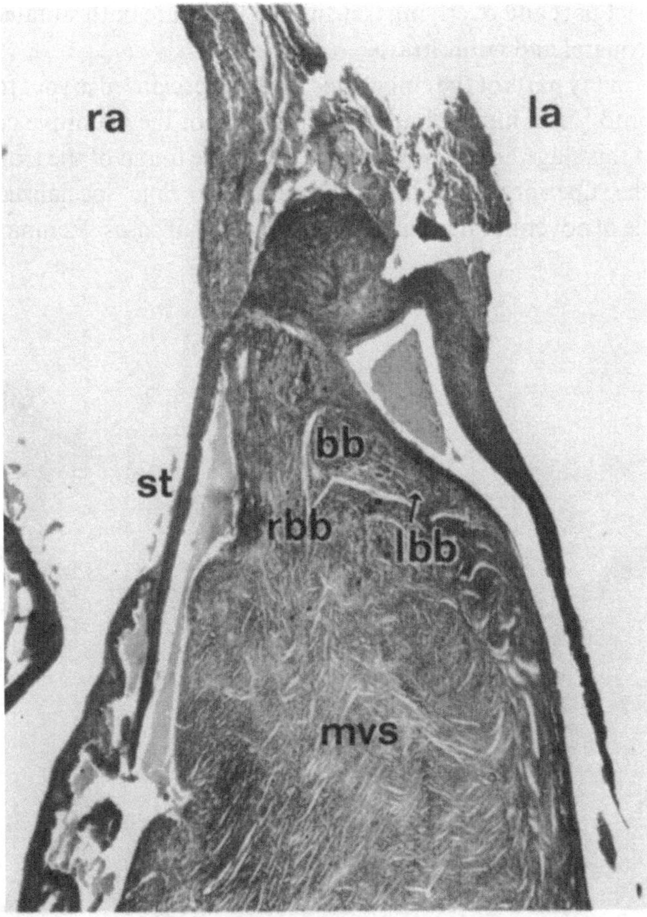

Figure 1. Frontal section through the septal part of the heart (human foetus, 230 mm C-R length). The branching bundle (bb) situated more to the left on the muscular ventricular septum (mvs), just divides into a right and a left bundle branch (rbb and lbb). A muscle column is present between the base of the septal leaflet of the tricuspid valve (st) and the bb. ra: right atrium; la: left atrium. Azan, 8×.

side a muscular column ascended to the base of the septal leaflet of the tricuspid valve, separating the branching bundle from the endocardium (fig. 1). Thus the right bundle branch is forced to penetrate the septal myocardium before reaching the trabecula septomarginalis. Once a symmetrical position of the branching bundle was seen and once a muscle column was found at the left side, forcing the left bundle branch to pass a short distance through the myocardium to reach its subendocardial position.

The penetrating bundle and the atrioventricular node, which is constituted of a compact part and overlying transitional fibres are both situated as in the normal neonatal and adult hearts.

Clearly, many parts of the embryonic rings of specialized myocardium have persisted into foetal life, and are the precursors of the definitive conducting system. At this stage however, no remnants can be found of the truncobulbar ring and the superior part of the bulboventricular ring. Specialized myocardium in the atrioventricular sulcus was found in all cases. Remnants of this

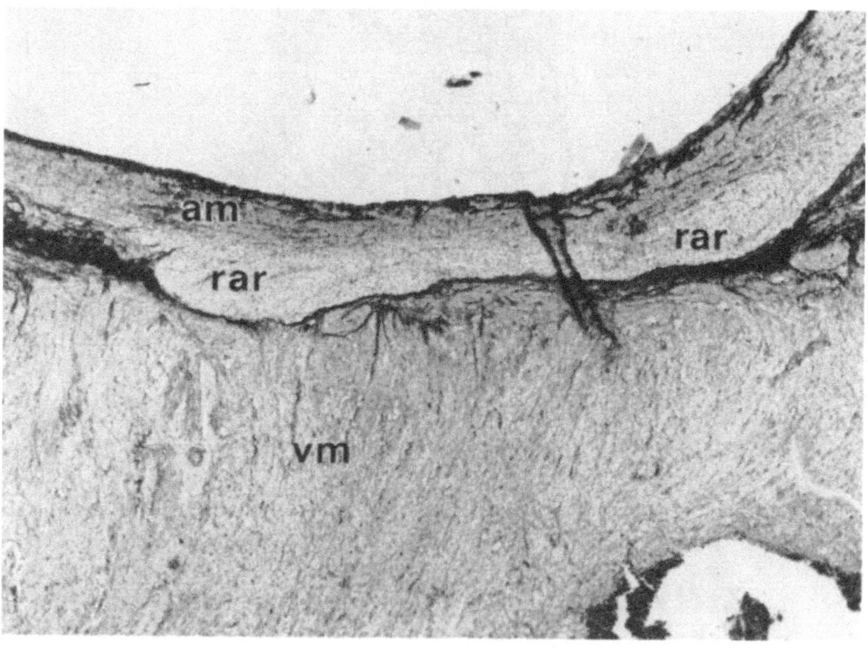

Figure 2. Section of the heart of a human foetus of 125 mm C-R length, showing the anterior part of the right atrioventricular ring (rar), which is paler than the overlying plain atrial myocardium (am). The fibrous anulus of the tricuspid orifice separating the rar from the ventricular myocardium (vm) is here very thin. resorcin fuchsin, picric acid, thiazin-red; 39.8 ×.

atrioventricular ring tissue may be found in the fully developed heart. The right atrioventricular ring could easily be recognized (fig. 2), whereas only parts of the left atrioventricular ring were seen. In some cases the left atrioventricular ring could no longer be detected.

The following observations are relevant to the fate of the sinuatrial ring, which gives rise to the sinuatrial node and contributes to the transitional fibres of the atrioventricular node. A complete sinuatrial ring comparable to, for instance, the right atrioventricular ring, was not seen. In two hearts, however, (table 1) tracts of pale cells were seen in the atrial septum. These cells could easily be differentiated from the overlying atrial myocardium, the former having a paler cytoplasm and often a somewhat more globular arrangement.

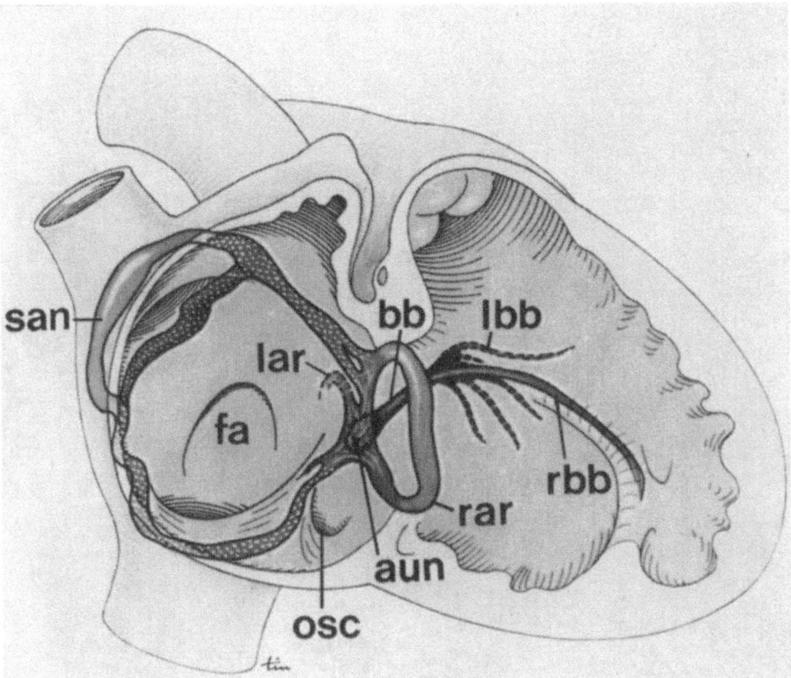

Figure 3. Graphic reconstruction of the specialized myocardium of the same heart as in fig. 2. lbb: left bundle branch; rbb: right bundle branch; bb: branching bundle; aun: atrioventricular node; rar: right atrioventricular ring; lar: left atrioventricular ring; san: sinuatrial node; fa: fossa ovalis; osc: ostium sinu coronarii. The tracts connecting the atrioventricular junctional area with the sinuatrial node are dotted.

In 4 of the remaining 7 cases pale cells were not found in the atrial septum or in the wall, 2 cases could not be studied in this respect as the lateral part of the heart had been removed, and in 1 case the staining technique was deficient.

The modified elastic tissue stain as performed in the hearts studied has been developed in our laboratory (4) and proved in general to be an excellent staining method for the study of the histology of the foetal heart.

A graphic reconstruction of the specialized myocardium with surrounding structures was made in case 5. The distribution of the tracts of pale cells was also indicated (fig. 3), they constitute a fibre to fibre continuity between the right atrioventricular ring close to the atrioventricular junctional area, and the sinuatrial node. This connection is effected by one branch passing behind and another in front of the superior caval vein. In this way the superior caval vein is encircled. The sinuatrial node is situated at the lateral margin of the

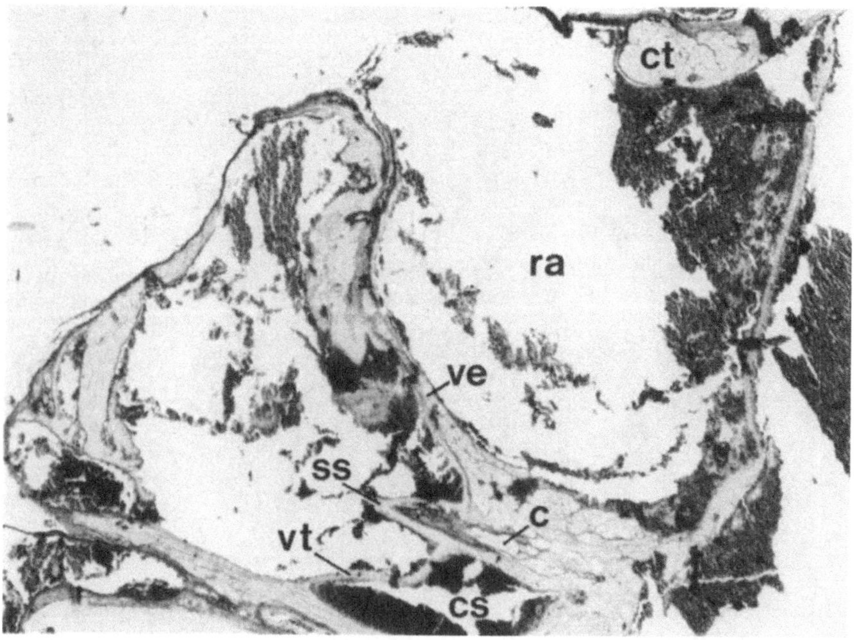

Figure 4. Section through the lateral part of the right atrium of the same heart as pictured in fig. 2 and 3. A group of pale coloured cells (c) is visible in the base of the right venous valve next to the coronary sinus (cs). vt: valvula Thebesii; ss: sinus septum; ve: valvula Eustachii. In a more posterior section the cells are continuous with a similar type of cells lying in the crista terminalis (ct) in this way connecting the atrioventricular junctional area with the sinuatrial node. resorcin-fuchsin, picric acid, thiazin red; 18.9×.

junction of the superior caval vein with the right atrium and has an extension along the crista terminalis. From this extension another tract of pale cells emanates and passes through the base of the right venous valve between the coronary sinus and the inferior caval vein, reaching the transitional fibres of the atrioventricular node in the region where the tendon of Todaro enters the Eustachian valve (fig. 4 and 5).

The transitional fibres of the atrioventricular node were evident in almost every case as an extension along the lateral side of the tendon of Todaro and thus lying outside the Koch triangle (see Anderson, this book, page 25).

Accessory connections of the compound part of the node and fasciculo-ventricular fibres as described by Anderson (7) were encountered in all of these foetal hearts connecting some parts of specialized tissue with plain ventricular myocardium (fig. 5).

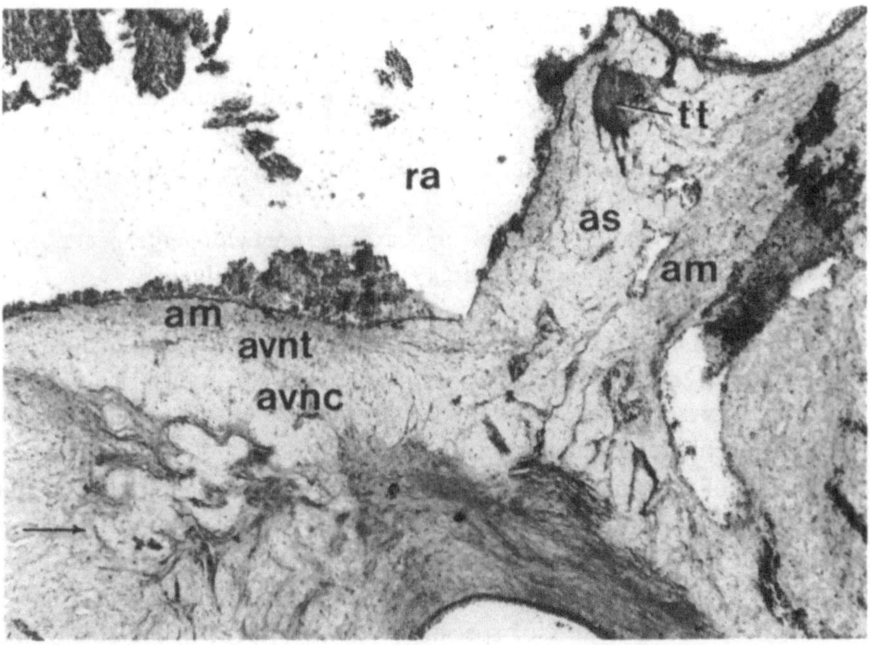

Figure 5. Section through the atrioventricular junctional area of the same heart as pictured in fig. 2, 3 and 4. Note the atrioventricular node with a compound part (avnc) and overlying transitional fibres (avnt). The transitional fibres ascend into the atrial septum (as) and surround the tendon of Todaro (tt). Plain atrial myocardium (am) is slightly darker in colour. Arrow: part of the specialized myocardium of the penetrating bundle is continuous with plain ventricular myocardium thus constituting an accessory connection. resorcin fuchsin, picric acid, thiazin red; 39.8 ×.

DISCUSSION

As is evident from the observations, the foetal condition constitutes an intermediate stage with respect to the amount of detectable specialized tissue, i.e. some parts of the embryonic rings are no longer detectable, but the configuration normally encountered in the adult has not yet been achieved.

The varying relationship between the branching bundle and the muscular ventricular septum may be found in the foetal as well as in the infant heart, as is evident from three neonatal specimens (unpublished observations) and from a recent paper (8). Our own observations (9) on the embryology of the conducting system make the embryological explanation by Baissus et al. (8), of this phenomenon, unlikely. We would suggest that the ventricular septum develops from several components which may have a varying relationship. The presence in some hearts of a postero-medial muscle is thought to be related to this problem (see Wenink, this book, page 129).

According to the literature (7) fasciculo-ventricular connections are features of most normal hearts, and this also applies to the accessory connections seen in these cases which are accessory nodoventricular muscle bundles from the compact node to the ventricular myocardium. There is a tendency in the latter group for them to diminish in number with increasing age and further development of the fibrous anuli.

Bypass tracts similar to atrial myocardium contacting the penetrating bundle, as described in the literature (7), were not encountered.

In accordance with the results of studies on foetal hearts performed by Anderson and Taylor (2) atrioventricular ring tissue was found in all specimens. In most cases the right atrioventricular ring was complete, whereas the left ring, if present at all, was only partial. The apparent dominance of the right atrioventricular ring has yet to be explained.

The fate of the sinuatrial ring, which gives rise to the sinuatrial node and contributes to the atrioventricular node deserves special attention. The exact position of this ring in the atrium is not known as the site of the left venous valve on the atrial septum is not distinct. The tracts of pale cells, found in two hearts, might be remnants of specialized tissue present in the embryonic period which normally disappear during further development, as do other parts of the embryonic ring tissues. The occasional finding of these tracts in the foetus does not of course prove the much disputed existence of internodal pathways in the adult. Critical analysis of literature data, concerning this subject, have been published recently (10). It is shown that the criteria for the existence of internodal pathways as laid down by Janse and Anderson (11) on the basis of their study of Aschoff (12) and Mönckeberg (13, 14) have not up to date been fulfilled. The existence of internodal pathways could only be confirmed histologically and then not satisfactorily in a few isolated cases (15, 1). In this respect these connections are obviously different from other constantly found parts of the conducting system present in fully developed hearts.

The distribution of internodal pathways shown, for instance, in a well-known atlas (16) bears a strong resemblance to the position of the tracts of pale cells in our reconstructed specimen. The alleged histological confirmation of the presence of internodal pathways in the adult heart might be based on the persistance of embryonic ring tissue in the atrium in some exceptional cases. This phenomenon is frequently seen with atrioventricular ring specialized myocardium.

Electrophysiologically, broad preferential routes in the atria do exist (see Tynan, this book, page 35). These routes coincide by and large with the pale tracts seen in our reconstruction.

Knowledge of the fate of those parts of the embryonic specialized myocardium that can no longer be recognized in the adult heart is essential for a better understanding of the above findings. Have these tissues changed into histologically normal working myocardium with or without preferential conducting capacities, or have they altogether disappeared?

REFERENCES

1. Robb, J. S. and Petri, R., Expansions of the atrioventricular system in the atria. In: Paes de Carvalho, A., de Mello, W. C. and Hoffman, B. F. (ed.), *The specialized tissue of the heart.* Amsterdam 1961.
2. Anderson, R. H. and Taylor, I. M., Development of atrioventricular specialized tissue in human heart. *Br. Heart. J.* 34, 1205 (1972).
3. Anderson, R. H., Davies, M. J. and Becker, A. E., Atrioventricular ring specialized tissue in the normal heart. *Eur. J. Cardiol.* 2, 219 (1974).
4. Hoefsmit, E. Chr. M., *Het sluitingsproces van de ductus arteriosus bij de rat.* Thesis Leiden 1967.
5. Anderson, R. H., Becker, A. E., Brechenmacher, C., Davies, M. J., Rossi, L., The human atrioventricular junctional area. *Eur. J. Cardiol.* 3, 11 (1975).
6. Becker, A. E. and Anderson, R. H., Morphology of the human atrioventricular junctional area. In: Wellens et al. (ed.), *The conducting system of the heart. Structure, function and clinical implications.* Leiden 1976.
7. Anderson, R. H., Becker, A. E., Brechenmacher, C., Davies, J. M., Rossi, L., Ventricular preexcitation. A proposed nomenclature for its substrates. *Eur. J. Cardiol.* 3, 27 (1975).
8. Baissus, C., Latour, H., Grolleau, R., Puech, P., Branche droite du faisceau de His. *Arch. Mal. Coeur* 11, 1123 (1976).

9. Wenink, A. C. G., Development of the human cardiac conducting system. *J. Anat.* 121, 617 (1976).
10. Chuaqui, B. J., Über die Ausbreitungsbündel des Sinusknotens. *Virchows Arch. Abt. A. Path. Anat.* 355, 179 (1971).
11. Janse, M. J. and Anderson, R. H., Specialized internodal atrial pathways – fact or fiction? *Eur. J. Cardiol.* 2, 117 (1974).
12. Aschoff, L., Referat über die Herzstörungen in ihren Beziehungen zu dem spezifischen Muskelsystem des Herzens. *Verh. Dtsch. Ges. Pathol.* 14, 3 (1910).
13. Mönckeberg, J. G., Beiträge zur normalen und pathologischen Anatomie des Herzens. *Verh. Dtsch. Ges. Pathol.* 14, 64 (1910).
14. Mönckeberg, J. G., Das spezifische Muskelsystem im menschlichen Herzen. *Ergebn. allg. Path. path. Anat.* 19, 328 (1924).
15. Thorel, C., Vorläufige Mitteilung über eine besondere Muskelverbindung zwischen der Cava superior und dem Hisschen Bündel. *Münch. Med. Wochenschr.* 56, 2159 (1909).
16. Hoffman, B. F. In: Yonkman, F. F. (ed.), *The Ciba Collection of Medical Illustrations, Vol. 5*, Section 1, plate 12. New York 1969.

3. THE MORPHOLOGY OF THE NORMAL CONDUCTING SYSTEM*

R. H. ANDERSON AND A. E. BECKER

INTRODUCTION

It is unfortunate that many recent accounts of the disposition and histology of the conducting tissues of the heart ignore the initial presentations of Tawara (1) and Keith and Flack (2), together with the expansions of this early work reported by Mönckeberg (3) and Koch (4). Our own studies have proved to be very much a restatement of this initial work. In this presentation these findings will be described.

a) The Sinuatrial Node

The sinuatrial node, or normal pacemaker of the heart, is a small, spindle shaped structure located in the sulcus terminalis (fig. 1). As indicated by Keith and Flack (2) and endorsed by subsequent workers (5, 6), the node is primarily a lateral structure relative to the sinuatrial junction. Although there is considerable individual variation, it is rare in our experience to find the node extending across the auricular crest, as suggested by Hudson (7). There is usually an extensive posterior prolongation of the node along the sulcus terminalis, the cauda, which frequently extends towards the orifice of the inferior vena cava. The node is a directly sub-epicardial structure, being located in the external junction of the wall of the superior vena cava and the crista terminalis (fig. 2). The cauda frequently runs intramyocardially before merging with the atrial myocardium (fig. 2b). Histologically the node is made up of interweaving small cells arranged in fasciculi and bound together in a dense fibrous tissue matrix. Although usually arranged around a central artery (fig. 2), there is marked individual variation, and it is frequent to find hearts with numerous small arteries ramifying in the nodal substance rather than possessing a single large artery. The artery of supply also shows variation in its course. It normally runs along the medial wall of the atrium and

* Supported in part by a grant from the British Heart Foundation.

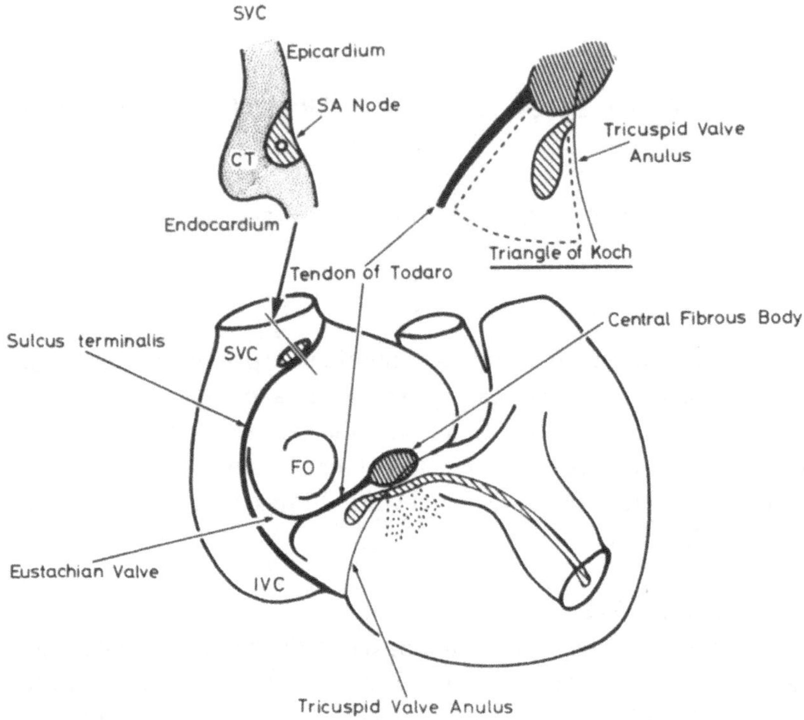

Figure 1. Diagram illustrating the gross landmarks to the sinuatrial (SA) node and the atrioventricular junctional area. (SVC: superior vena cava; IVC: inferior vena cava; FO: foramen ovale; CT: crista terminalis)

may then pass in front of, behind or may divide so as to encircle the orifice of the superior vena cava.

At the margins of the node where it abuts against atrial myocardium, the nodal cells merge rapidly on all sides with the atrial myocardial cells, the transitional zone being abrupt. We have been unable to identify tracts of specialized tissue extending from the sinuatrial node into the atrial septum (vide infra).

b) The Internodal Atrial Myocardium

Controversy has existed for many years regarding the nature of the internodal atrial myocardium (8). It is pertinent to remember that the bundle described by Wenckebach himself (9) connected the musculature of the superior vena cava and the right atrium, and was reported *prior* to the discovery of the

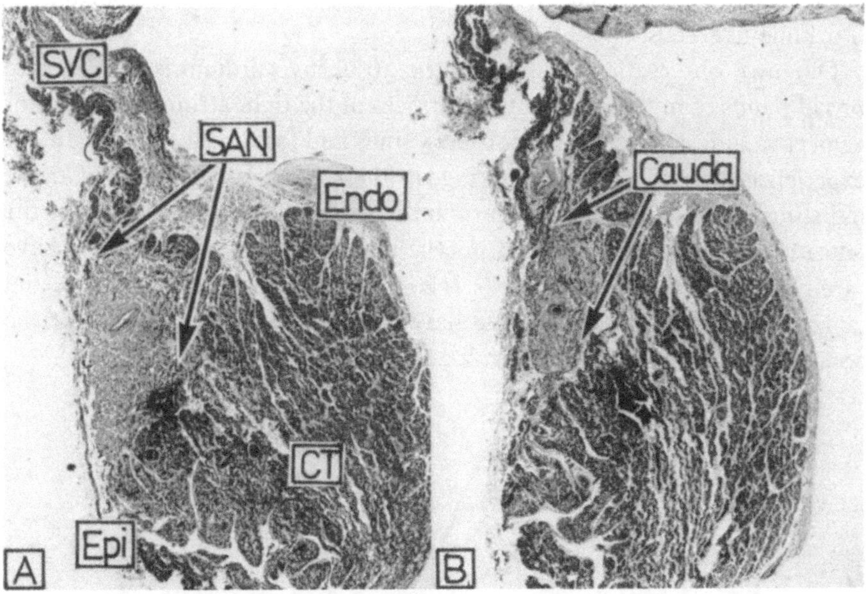

Figure 2. Histological section through the sinuatrial node of a neonatal heart. Figure 2A is through the body of the node (SAN) which is a triangular structure located at the epicardial (Epi) junction of the superior vena cava (SVC) with the crista terminalis (CT). Note that the node is arranged around a central artery. Endo-endocardium. Figure 2B is a section through the cauda of the node, which has turned intramyocardially just prior to merging with the myocardium of the posterior atrial wall.

sinuatrial node. The bundle described by Bachmann (10) was discovered using only physiological techniques, Bachmann himself suggesting that the rapid conduction was a consequence of the alignment of the myocardial fibers. Thorel (11) was the first to suggest that a bundle of 'Purkinje' fibers extended from the sinus node, and this proposition was debated at length by the German Pathological Society (12). The consensus of this meeting was that histologically differentiated tracts were lacking in the internodal atrial tissues. Mönckeberg (3) and Aschoff (13) subsequently made the suggestion that workers describing specialized tracts in the atria should satisfy certain criteria, namely that the cells of the tract be histologically discrete from the atrial myocardium and that the purported tract be isolated by fibrous tissue from the remainder of the atrial septum. It is evident that subsequent proponents of specialized tracts (14-16) have never suggested that the tracts are isolated from the remainder of the atrial myocardium. Specialization has been suggested on the basis that the purported tracts contain a proportion of 'Purkinje-like' cells.

Our own observations show that the atrial myocardium is divided into broad bands of myocardium by the orifices of the right atrium, the superior vena cava, inferior vena cava, coronary sinus and fossa ovalis (fig. 3). In our experience, the myocardium making up these band is composed of tissue indistinguishable from the myocardium of the right atrial appendage or the left atrium. In the infantile and puerile material we have studied we have rarely observed 'Purkinje-like' cells. It is our opinion that the internodal atrial myocardium is unspecialized. We have found *no* evidence to support the concept of morphologically specialized internodal pathways.

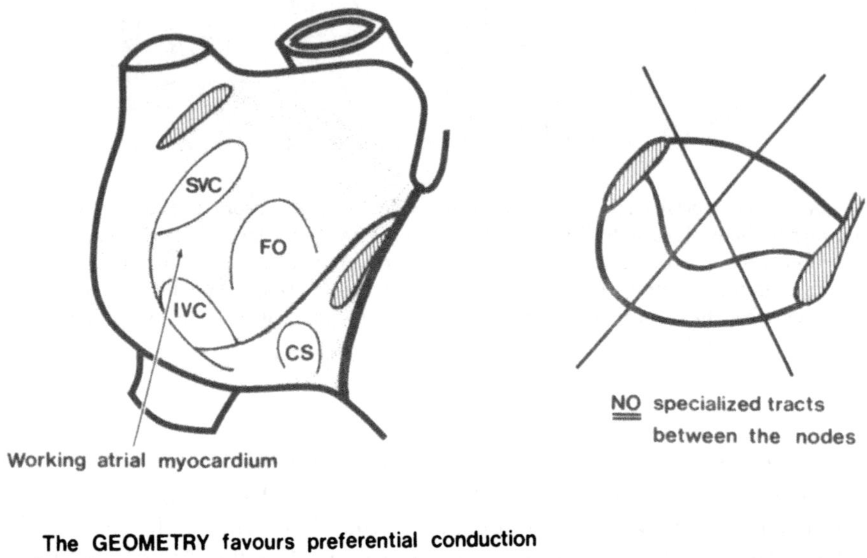

Figure 3. Diagrams illustrating the nature of the internodal atrial myocardium. Our findings show that there are *no* specialized tracts in the interatrial septum or crista terminalis. SVC: superior vena cava; IVC: inferior vena cava; CS: coronary sinus; FO: foramen ovale.

c) The Atrioventricular Junctional Area

The gross landmarks of the atrioventricular junctional area were well described by Koch (4). He pointed out that a triangle could be constructed between the anulus of the tricuspid valve, the continuation of the Eustachian valve into the central fibrous body (the tendon of Todaro) and the orifice of the coronary sinus. The site of the penetrating atrioventricular bundle is at the

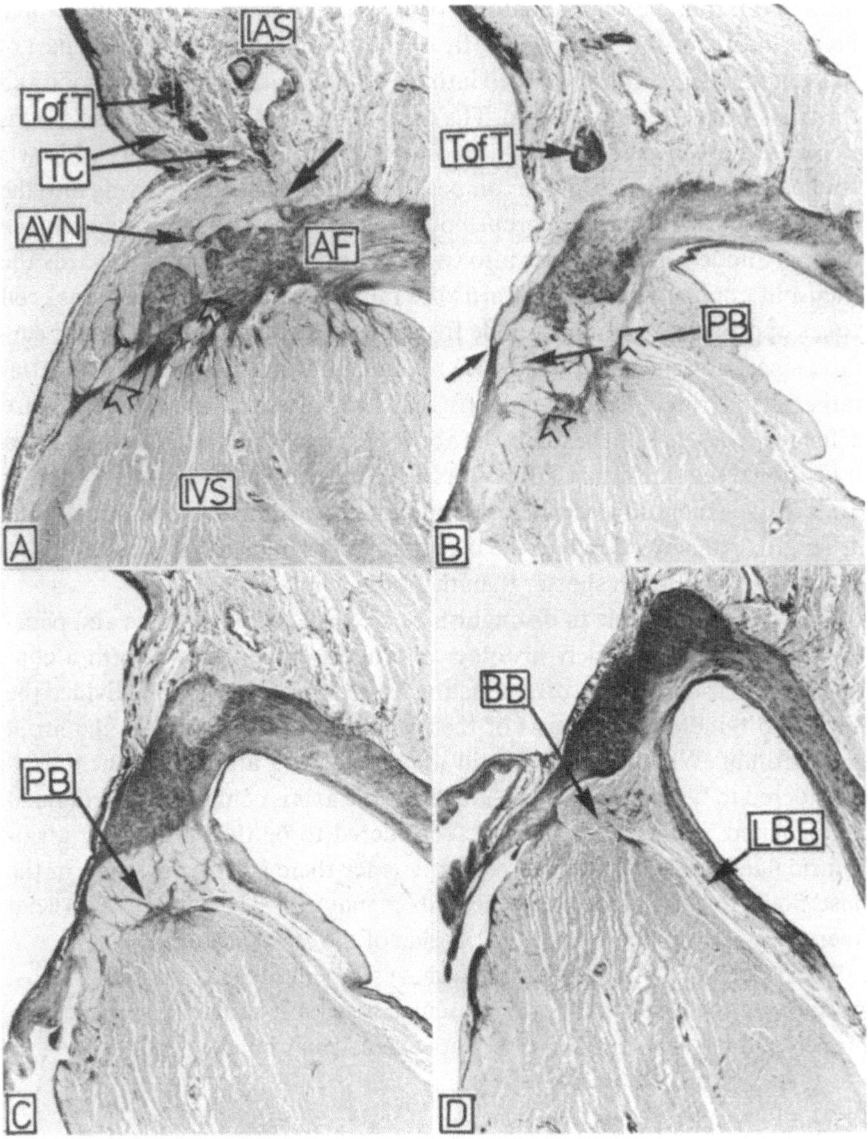

Figure 4. Histological sections through the atrioventricular junctional area of a neonatal heart. Figure 4A is through the node. Note that the compact node (AVN) is an interatrial structure, being connected by short transitional cells (TC) to the superficial and deep parts of the interatrial septum (IAS). Note also the extensions from the node (open arrows) into the anulus fibrosus (AF). IVS: interventricular septum. T of T: Tendon of Todaro. Figure 4B shows the point at which the compact node becomes the penetrating bundle (PB). It is the point at which the nodal–bundle axis ceases to make contact with the atrial tissues (closed arrow). Note the connexions between the bundle and the crest of the septum (open arrows). Figure 4C shows the penetrating bundle astride the muscular septum. Figure 4D shows the commencement of the branching bundle (BB), the left bundle branch fibers (LBB) streaming down as a fan-like sheet.

apex of this triangle, and the entirety of the atrial component of the junctional area is located within the triangle (fig. 1). Histologically (17) the atrial part of the junctional area can be divided into the compact atrioventricular node and the transitional cell zone (fig. 4). The compact node is adherent to the anulus fibrosus, and clings to the anulus along its length. In the majority of hearts studied by us extensions of the compact node are observed ramifying into the fibrous anulus and central fibrous body (fig. 4). When traced posteriorly the compact node usually divides into two extensions, one running towards the tricuspid anulus, the other towards the mitral anulus. The transitional cell zones approach the compact node from all sides apart from the anular surface, since, as Scherf and Cohen (18) pointed out, the node is an *inter*atrial rather than a right atrial structure (fig. 4). The posterior transitional cells are extensive, passing both beneath and above the coronary sinus. The right sided transitional cells are divided into superficial and deep groups by the tendon of Todaro. The more superficial fibers run across the compact node throughout its length, extending down to the tricuspid valve anulus. The left sided transitional cells are much shorter than the right.

We have been unable to distinguish between the compact node and penetrating bundle using solely histological criteria, since the two form a continuous nodal-bundle axis of conducting tissue. We have therefore divided the node and bundle on the basis of the insulation of the axis from the atrial myocardium. While the axis is still in contact with atrial cells, the axis is considered to be compact node. As soon as the axis is completely surrounded and isolated by fibrous tissue, it is considered to be the penetrating atrioventricular bundle (fig. 4b). In our experience there is wide variation in the 'last' fibers to contact the axis. These fibers may either be overlay superficial fibers or else deep fibers from the left side of the atrial septum.

The penetrating bundle is usually a short segment of the nodal-bundle axis. As soon as the axis reaches the muscular septum it usually commences to branch and becomes the branching atrioventricular bundle (fig. 5).

d) The Ventricular Conducting Tissues

There is a marked difference in morphology of the right and left bundle branches. The right bundle branch is a narrow cord-like structure usually composed of myocardium little differentiated from the working myocardium (fig. 5). It usually runs intramyocardially and can be traced through the substance of the trabecula septomarginalis towards the moderator band, where it ramifies amongst the right ventricular myocardium. In contrast, the left bundle branch is an extensive sheet of cells running down the smooth left

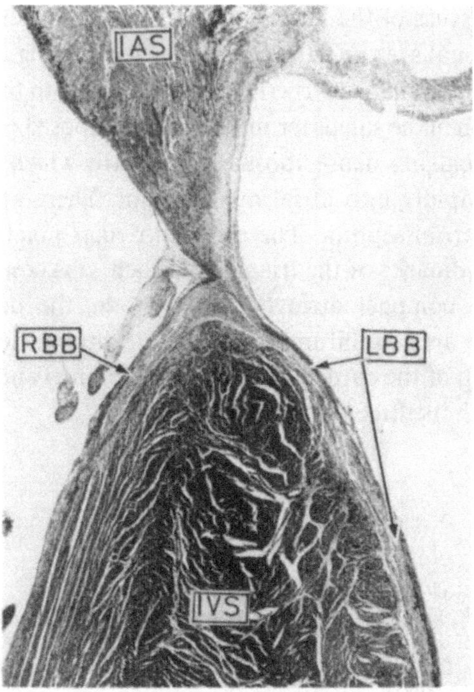

Figure 5. Histological section of the anterior part of the bifurcation from an adolescent heart. The left bundle branch is a sheet of cells (compare with Figure 4D) but the right bundle branch is a thin cord-like structure.

side of the interventricular septum (fig. 5). The initial part of the bundle is a continuous fan. As the branch descends the septum it radiates, usually producing three interconnected divisions as initially described by Tawara (1) and subsequently endorsed by others (19-21). In our experience it is exceedingly rare to find morphological division of the left bundle into two divisions alone; instead an anterior, middle and posterior division are usually found. It is also rare to find 'Purkinje' cells in the bundle branches of infantile hearts. The cells are somewhat larger than myocardial cells in the left bundle branch, but of similar size in the right bundle. Nonetheless, in both branches they are insulated from the septal surface. Large, vacuolated cells such as found in ungulate hearts are not found normally to compose the human ventricular conducting tissues.

SUMMARY

The conducting tissues of the heart comprise the sinuatrial node, the atrioventricular junctional area and the ventricular conducting tissues. The sinuatrial node is a spindle shaped structure situated lateral to the superior caval-right atrial junction in the sulcus terminalis. It is composed of small cells set in interweaving fasciculi in a dense fibrous tissue matrix which at the margins of the node merge rapidly into atrial myocardium. There are no specialized tracts within the atrial septum. The atrioventricular junctional area is delineated by the landmarks of the triangle of Koch. It is composed of a transitional zone, the compact atrioventricular node, the penetrating atrioventricular bundle and the bifurcating bundle. The ventricular conducting tissues are made up of the cord-like right bundle branch and the fan-like left bundle branch with its three terminal divisions.

REFERENCES

1. Tawara, S., *Das Reizleitungssystem des Säugetierherzens.* Jena 1906.
2. Keith, A. and Flack, M. W., The form and nature of the muscular connections between the primary divisions of the vertebrate heart. *J. Anat. Physiol.* 41, 171 (1907).
3. Mönckeberg, J. G., Das spezifische Muskelsystem im menschlichen Herzen. *Ergebn. allg. Pathol. Anat.* 19, 328 (1921).
4. Koch, W., *Der funktionelle Bau des menschlichen Herzens.* Urban u. Schwarzenberg, Berlin 1922 pp 92-102.
5. James, T. N., Anatomy of the human sinus node. *Anat. Rec.* 141, 109 (1961).
6. Truex, R. C., Smythe, M. Q. and Taylor, M. J., Reconstruction of the human sinuatrial node. *Anat. Rec.* 159, 371 (1967).
7. Hudson, R. E. B., The human pacemaker and its pathology. *Br. Heart J.* 22, 153 (1960).
8. Janse, M. J. and Anderson R. H., Specialized internodal atrial pathways – fact or fiction? *Eur. J. Cardiol.* 2, 117 (1974).
9. Wenckebach, K. F., Beiträge zur Kenntnis der menschlichen Herztätigkeit. *Arch. Anat. Physiol.* 2, 1 (1907).
10. Bachmann, G., The inter-auricular time interval. *Am. J. Physiol.* 41, 309 (1916).
11. Thorel, C., Vorläufige Mitteilung über eine besondere Muskelverbindung zwischen der Cava superior und dem Hisschen Bündel. *Münch. Med. Wochenschr.* 56, 2159 (1909).
12. Bericht über die Verhandlungen der XIV Tagung der Deutschen pathologischen Gesellschaft in Erlangen vom 4-6 april, *Zentralbl. Allg. Pathol.* 21, 433 (1910).
13. Aschoff, L., Referat über die Herzstörungen in ihren Beziehungen zu dem spezifischen Muskelsystem des Herzens. *Verh. Dtsch. Ges. pathol.* 14, 3 (1910).
14. Condorelli, L., Über die Bahnen der Reizleitung vom Keith-Flackschen Knoten zu den Vorhofen. *Z. ges. exp. Med.* 68, 493 (1929).
15. Franco, M., Recherches sur les faisceaux de connexion auriculaires dans les conditions normales et pathologiques. *Arch. Mal. Coeur* 44, 289 (1951).
16. James, T. N., The connecting pathways between the sinus node and the A-V node and between the right and left atrium in the human heart. *Am. Heart J.* 66, 498 (1963).

17. Becker, A. E. and Anderson, R. H., Morphology of the human atrioventricular junctional area. In: *The Conduction System of the Heart – Structure, Function and Clinical Implications.* Ed. Wellens, H. J. J., Lie, K. I. and Janse, M. J. Leiden 1976 p. 263.
18. Scherf, D. and Cohen, J., *The Atrioventricular Node and Selected Arrhythmias.* New York, p. V, 1964.
19. Rossi, L., Histopathology of the conducting system. *G. Ital. Cardiol.* 2, 484 (1972).
20. Kulbertus, H. E., The concept of left hemiblocks revisted. A histopathological and experimental study. *Adv. Cardiol.* 14, 126 (1975).
21. Massing, G. L. and James, T. N., Anatomical configuration of the His bundle and bundle branches in the human heart. *Circulation*, 53, 609 (1976).

4. INTERNODAL CONDUCTION PATHWAYS: SPECIALIZED OR PREFERENTIAL?

M. J. TYNAN

For many years there has been a controversy concerning the existence or non-existence of specialized tracts of fast conducting fibres which directly connect the sinuatrial (SA) and atrioventricular (AV) nodes. From the outset the question was whether the propagation of the wave of atrial activation was uniform as has been inferred from the work of Lewis et al. (1, 2, 3, 4) or whether it was faster in certain parts of the atria (5, 6, 7, 8). If atrial activation is non-uniform, then we have to ask, is this due to the presence of 'specialized' tracts of fast conducting fibres or merely to preferential routes of conduction in plain atrial myocardium? The historical background to the controversy which exists today has been well reviewed by Janse and Anderson (9). Discussion will therefore be concentrated on recent publications on the subject.

UNIFORM OR NON-UNIFORM ATRIAL ACTIVATION?

Detailed endocardial and epicardial mapping studies of the right atrium and endocardial studies of the right side of the interatrial septum (9, 10, 11) have demonstrated that atrial excitation is non-uniform. These studies involving the rabbit, the dog and man are all in basic agreement that the wave of activation passes more rapidly along the crista terminalis and the anterior part of the atrial septum than through other parts of the atrium.

SPECIALIZED OR PREFERENTIAL CONDUCTION

The consensus that atrial activation is propagated in a non-uniform manner is not associated with a similar consensus on the anatomical or physiological nature of the more rapid routes of conduction. Thorel (12, 13, 14) proposed the existence of a tract of specialized conducting tissue within the atria and more recently James and his colleagues (15, 16, 17) have championed the view that the sinuatrial and atrioventricular nodes are directly interconnected by several such tracts (fig. 1). They postulate that there are three internodal tracts, the anterior and middle ones being in the anterior part of the interatrial septum while the posterior one descends in the crista terminalis, crossing to the AV node via the region of the sinus septum. However, since the first suggestion of their presence, the existence of these tracts has been doubted. The two main approaches to the investigation of the problem are anatomical and electrophysiological. Both require precise definitions of the phenomena which must be observed to demonstrate the existence of specialized tracts.

Anatomical Evidence

The essential anatomical features of specialized tracts were summarized by Janse and Anderson (9) from the definitions of Aschoff (18) and Mönckeberg (19); to qualify as a specialized internodal tract there must be a continuous bundle of specialized cells, showing fibre to fibre continuity, connecting the SA and AV nodes; in addition, these tracts must be separated from the atrial myocardium by a sheath of connective tissue. Such tracts have never been

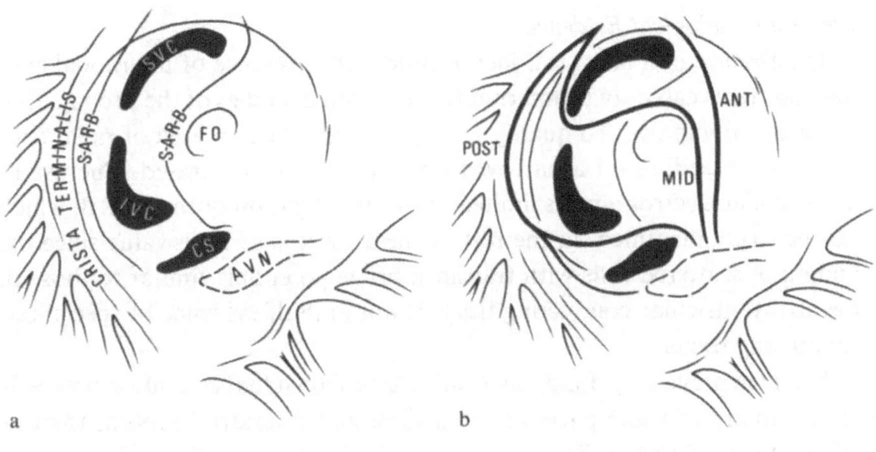

Figure 1. a: shows a schematic representation of the rabbit right atrium and atrial septum. SVC = superior vena cava, IVC = inferior vena cava, AVN = atrioventricular node, FO = foramen ovale, SARB = sinuatrial ring bundle. b: shows the proposed routes of specialized internodal tracts. ANT = anterior tract, MID = middle tract, POST = posterior tract. This last tract is said to pass through the region of the sinus septum but in the rabbit there are said to be a few fibres running inferiorly to the inferior vena cava. After James and Sherf, Am. J. Cardiol., 28: 414, 1971 and Merideth and Titus, Circulation, 37: 566, 1968.

identified in the atria. James and Sherf (15, 16, 17) have seen cells which they describe as 'specialized' interspersed with plain atrial cells, these alone are not sufficient to qualify as specialized tracts since they are not continuous and have no sheath. In fact, some of these cells may not have been specialized at all but may have been 'intercalated clear cells' which are probably artefactual (20). There is thus no convincing anatomical evidence for the existence of specialized internodal tracts. At this point, mention should be made of the sinuatrial ring bundle (SARB). This is a tract of cells running from the region of the SA node to the vicinity of the AV node, although not directly connecting to it (fig. 1). The cells in this bundle are not Purkinje cells but rather resemble small atrial cells. If the SARB is to be considered a specialized conducting pathway, confirmatory electrophysiological evidence is necessary (see below).

Elsewhere in this volume (page 15), Gittenberger-de Groot and Wenink have reported the finding in two embryos, of a tract of pale cells connecting the SA and AV nodes coursing through the atrial septum. Neither the nature nor the function of this tract is clear. At present these are isolated embryological observations whose relevance to internodal conduction in the mature heart has yet to be established.

Electrophysiological Evidence

In the absence of anatomical identification, the presence of internodal conducting tracts can only be inferred from mapping studies of the propagation of the atrial impulse. To qualify as a specialized tract an area of rapid conduction proceeding on a narrow front must be demonstrated. The use of intracellular electrograms is limited to the investigation of the SARB, which can be easily identified, in the rest of the atria it is of little value since the finding of scattered cells with transmembrane potentials similar to those in the atrioventricular conducting tissue is not in itself evidence of specialized conducting tracts.

As stated previously, mapping studies have shown that activation proceeds more rapidly in some parts of the atrium and interatrial septum than in others. Figure 2 shows diagrammatically the isochronous lines of activation found in the rabbit right atrium and atrial septum in two studies (9, 10). The waves of activation pass more rapidly down the crista terminalis and the anterior margin of the septum. The fossa ovalis is an 'obstruction' to propagation which is bypassed by the anterior and posterior routes. However, activation proceeds along broad fronts, not the narrow ones to be expected if conduction was by specialized tracts. During operations for transposition of

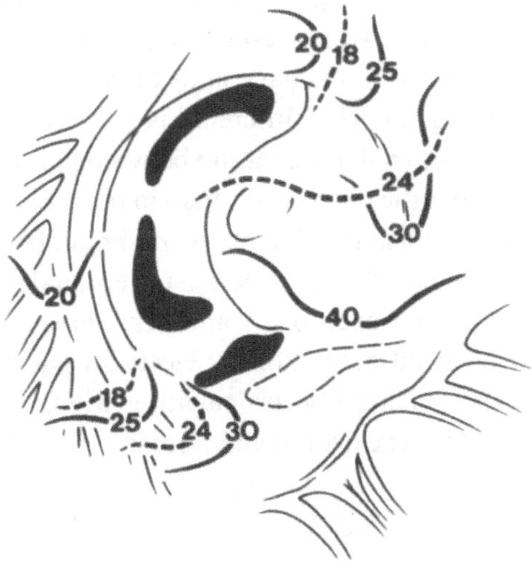

Figure 2. This shows the results of two mapping studies of atrial activation in the rabbit, showing isochronous lines of atrial activation (time in msc.) proceeding on broad fronts. After Spach et al., Circ. Res., 29: 157, 1971, and Janse and Anderson, Eur. J. Cardiol., 2: 117, 1974.

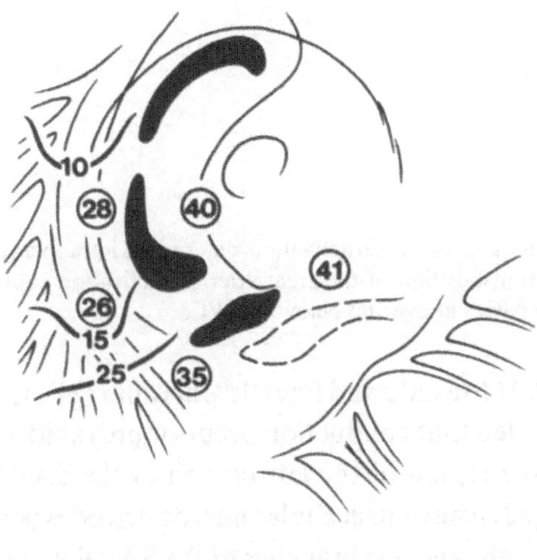

Figure 3. This shows the result of an endocardial mapping study, in solid lines, performed in the region of the SARB and a microelectrode study, in open circles, the electrodes impaling the right and left branches of the SARB and neighbouring plain atrial myocardium. Both studies show that the SARB conducts more slowly than the plain myocardium. After Masuda and Paes de Carvalho, Circ. Res., 37: 414, 1975, and Hiraoka and Sano, Am. J. Physiol., 231: 319. 1976.

the great arteries Wittig and colleagues (11) demonstrated a similar pattern of atrial activation in man (fig. 4), however, the posterior route passed both superiorly and inferiorly to the coronary sinus rather than inferiorly only as observed in the rabbit (fig. 2). This difference is presumably due to the fact that, in man, there is more atrial musculature between the coronary sinus and the superior vena cava and the fossa ovalis than in the rabbit. But in man, the rabbit and the dog (10) atrial activation occurs on broad fronts and proceeds most rapidly via muscle bundles like the crista terminalis where the plain atrial fibres are orientated parallel to one another. Furthermore, alterations in the site of origin of atrial activation by electrical pacing (9, 11) causes changes in the sequence of impulse propagation which suggest that conduction is via plain atrial myocardium and not via specialized pathways.

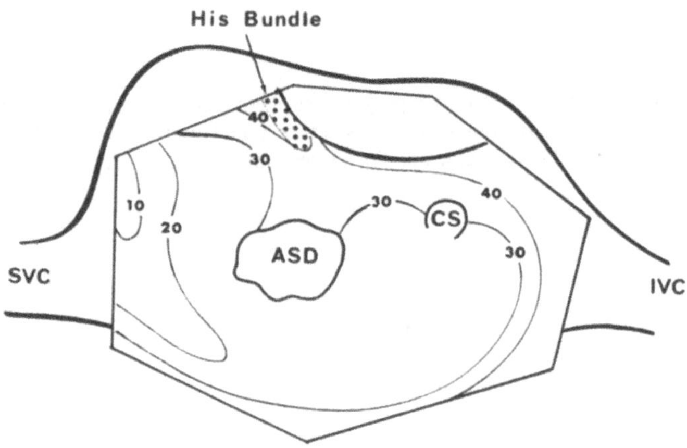

Figure 4. This shows the sequence of atrial activation, determined intraoperatively by Wittig et al. (1977) in patients with transposition of the great arteries. Activation is propagated on broad fronts but in the human passes above and below the IVC.

What of the SARB? Masuda and Paes de Carvalho (21), using endocardial mapping, demonstrated that conduction occurs more rapidly along the crista terminalis than in the region of the left branch of the SARB (fig. 3). Also, Hiraoka and Sano (22) using intracellular microelectrodes demonstrated that conduction in both right and left branches of the SARB was slower than that through the neighbouring atrial myocardium. Furthermore, they showed that cutting the SARB did not affect conduction from the SA to the AV node. Thus, the SARB is certainly not a specialized fast conducting tract nor is it important in internodal conduction.

Not only is atrial impulse propagation along routes with broad fronts but in the rabbit the posterior route leads to a posterior atrioventricular nodal input which is inferior to the coronary sinus and not via the sinus septum. In other words, in the rabbit the posterior input does not traverse the proposed route of the main component of the posterior internodal tract.

CONCLUSION

Although propagation of the wave of activation through the atrium is not uniform, there is general acceptance that it occurs on broad fronts along atrial muscle bundles. In these bundles the plain atrial myocardial cells are organized in a parallel fashion facilitating conduction along the long axis of the bundle. In no way can these bundles be considered specialized conducting tracts since this would mean that the whole of the anterior part of the septum would be such a tract. To use the term specialized internodal conducting tract in this sense is meaningless. In addition to the absence of experimental evidence for direct specialized internodal connexions, teleology would not lead us to reason that such tracts should exist. Rapid conduction of the impulse from the sinuatrial to the atrioventricular node, at velocities similar to those seen in the bundle of His, would necessitate an even longer atrioventricular nodal delay than is observed to occur (23), otherwise a significant part of atrial systole could occur during the onset of ventricular systole and thus the booster effect of atrial systole would be lost.

Despite the fact that specialized internodal connections do not exist, there are in the atria routes of preferential conduction occurring in plain atrial myocardium and awareness of their existence is probably of surgical importance.

REFERENCES

1. Lewis, T., Oppenheimer, B. S. and Oppenheimer, A., Site and origin of the mammalian heart beat: the pacemaker in the dog. *Heart* 2, 147 (1910).
2. Lewis, T., Meakins, J. and White, P. D., The excitatory process in the dog's heart, Part I – The auricles. *Phil. Trans. Roy. Soc. B.* 205, 375 (1914).
3. Lewis, T. In: Hoeber, P. H. (ed.), *Lectures on the Heart.* London 1915.
4. Lewis, T., *The mechanism and graphic registration of the heart beat.* London 1925.
5. Eyster, J. A. E. and Meek, W. J., Experiments on the origin and conduction of the impulse of the heart. Point of primary negativity in the mammalian heart and the spread of negativity to other regions. *Heart* 5, 119 (1914).

6. Eyster, J. A. E. and Meek, W. J., Experiments on the origin and conduction of the cardiac impulse. VI: Conduction of the excitation from the sino-auricular node to the right auricle and the auriculo-ventricular node. *Arch. Intern. Med.* 18, 775 (1916).
7. Eyster, J. A. E. and Meek, W. J., Origin and conduction of the heart beat. *Physiol. Rev.* 1, 1 (1921).
8. Eyster, J. A. E. and Meek, W. J., Experiments on the origin and conduction of the heart beat. IX: Sino-ventricular conduction. *Am. J. Physiol.* 61, 130 (1922).
9. Janse, M. J. and Anderson, R. H., Specialized internodal atrial pathways – fact or fiction? *Eur. J. Cardiol.* 2, 117 (1974).
10. Spach, M. S., Lieberman, M., Scott, J. G., Barr, R. C., Johnson, E. A. and Kootsey, J. M., Excitation sequences of the atrial septum and the AV node in isolated hearts of the dog and rabbit. *Circ. Res.* 29, 157 (1971).
11. Wittig, J. H., de Laval, M. R. and Stark, J., Intraoperative mapping of atrial activation before, during, and after the Mustard operation *J. Thorac. Cardiovasc. Surg.* 73, 1 (1977).
12. Thorel, C., Vorlaüfige Mitteilung über eine besondere Muskelverbindung zwischen der Cava superior und dem Hisschen Bündel. *Münch. Med Wochenschr.* 56, 2159 (1909).
13. Thorel, C., Über den Aufbau des Sinusknotens und seine Verbindung mit der Cava superior und dem Wenckebachschen Bündel. *Münch. Med Wochenschr.* 57, 183 (1910).
14. Thorel, C., Über die supraventrikularen Abschnitt des sog. Reizleitungssystem. *Verh. Dtsch. Ges. Pathol.* 14, 71 (1910).
15. James, T. N., Connecting pathways between the sinus node and AV node and between the right and left atrium in the human heart. *Am. Heart. J.* 66, 498 (1963).
16. James, T. N., Anatomy of the cardiac conduction system in the rabbit. *Circ. Res.* 20, 638 (1967).
17. James, T. N. and Sherf, L., Specialized tissues and preferential conduction in the atria of the heart. *Am. J. Cardiol.* 28, 414 (1971).
18. Aschoff, L., Referat über die Herzstörungen in ihren Beziehungen zu dem spezifischen Muskelsystem des Herzens. *Verh. Dtsch. Ges. Pathol.* 14, 3 (1910).
19. Mönckeberg, J. G., Beiträge zur normalen und pathologischen Anatomie des Herzens. *Verh. Dtsch. Ges. Pathol.* 14, 64 (1910).
20. Tranum-Jensen, J., The fine structure of the atrial and atrioventricular junctional specialized tissues of the rabbit heart. In: Wellens et al. (ed.), *The conduction system of the heart.* Leiden 1976.
21. Masuda, M. O. and Paes de Carvalho, A., Sinuatrial transmission and atrial invasion during normal rhythm in the rabbit heart. *Circ. Res.* 37, 414 (1975).
22. Hiraoka, M. and Sano, T., Role of the sinuatrial ring bundle in internodal conduction. *Am. J. Physiol.* 231, 319 (1976).
23. Tynan, M., The function of specialized conducting tissue in the atria. *Med. Hypoth.* 1, 128 (1975).

PART I

CONDUCTING SYSTEM

B. Disposition in congenital heart malformations

5. THE CONDUCTING TISSUES IN CONGENITALLY COMPLETE HEART BLOCK, A CLINICO-PATHOLOGIC CORRELATION IN THREE PATIENTS

A. E. BECKER, T. G. LOSEKOOT AND R. H. ANDERSON

INTRODUCTION

Whilst congenitally complete heart block is known to occur frequently in congenitally malformed hearts, it can also occur in an otherwise normal structured heart (1, 2). In the latter situation, histological studies have always demonstrated a developmental error in the formation of the atrioventricular conduction system. Lev and his colleagues (1, 3-6), on the basis of their studies, have proposed a division of congenitally complete heart block into two basic varieties, firstly hearts in which atrial myocardium does not contact specialized conduction tissues, and secondly hearts in which an interruption is present within the nodal-bundle axis, the more proximal parts of the atrioventricular junctional area having developed normally.

Embryological studies of the atrioventricular conduction tissues have shown that this system develops *in situ*, albeit from different anlagen (7-9). For instance, the transitional cell zone forms most probably from the inferior limbus of the developing atrial septum, while the compact node forms from a posterior invagination of specialized atrioventricular ring tissues, probably dependant upon normal development of the posterior segment of the interventricular septum. The distal parts of the atrioventricular conduction system develop within the ventriculo-bulbar loop, possibly from specialized ventriculo-bulbar ring tissue. In order to form a continuous axis of atrioventricular conduction tissues it is necessary to have fusion of these segments. This is a crucial developmental phenomenon since in order to fuse the two anlagen must be juxtaposed, this process depending on a normal septation process within the heart. The abnormal disposition of the atrioventricular conduction system in, for example, univentricular hearts relates to lack of such juxtaposition. Moreover, in order to establish a continuous conduction axis it is also necessary for the sheath of embryonic connective tissue that normally envelops the specialized ring tissues to dissolve at the site of fusion between the two anlagen. This embryonic connective tissue, the so-called sulcus tissue, is of further interest since it will in part differentiate into the definitive anulus fibrosus, through which the conduction axis will then 'penetrate' to reach the ventricular myocardium (10).

Thus, it can be suggested that from a developmental point of view the atrioventricular conduction system is of 'segmental' origin. Pathologic specimens thusfar examined support this concept by revealing 'segmental' aberrations. Our own experiences with three patients with congenitally complete heart block, previously described in detail elsewhere (10), further endorse these concepts.

REPORT OF PATIENTS

Since the data concerning these three patients have been reported extensively in a previous communication (10), we will limit ourselves here to a brief outline of the most relevant features.

Patient 1

This baby girl was born spontaneously at term, following an uncomplicated pregnancy. The diagnosis of congenitally complete heart block was suspected immediately after birth because of a slow heart rate and a characteristic electrocardiogram (fig. 1). The atrial rate was 150 per minute and the ventricular rate 50 per minute. The ECG showed peaked P-waves and narrow QRS complexes, the morphology of the latter suggesting a high left-sided origin of the ventricular pacemaker. Cardiac catheterization studies, revealed isthmal hypoplasia, a large patent ductus arteriosus, an atrial septal defect and equal systolic pressures in right and left ventricles, with an intact ventricular septum.

The child initially improved with a treatment of digoxin and diuretics, but progressive vomiting made an intravenous drip necessary. The ventricular rate decreased to 40 beats per minute for which aleudrine was administered. The baby nevertheless died at the age of 18 days.

The autopsy confirmed the clinical diagnosis of a basically normally constructed heart, albeit with an atrial septal defect, isthmal hypoplasia and patent ductus arteriosus. For histopathologic investigation of the atrioventricular conduction system a tissue block was removed which encompassed the entirety of the inter-atrial septum, including the ostia of the superior and inferior caval veins, the origin of the aorta, the crista supraventri-

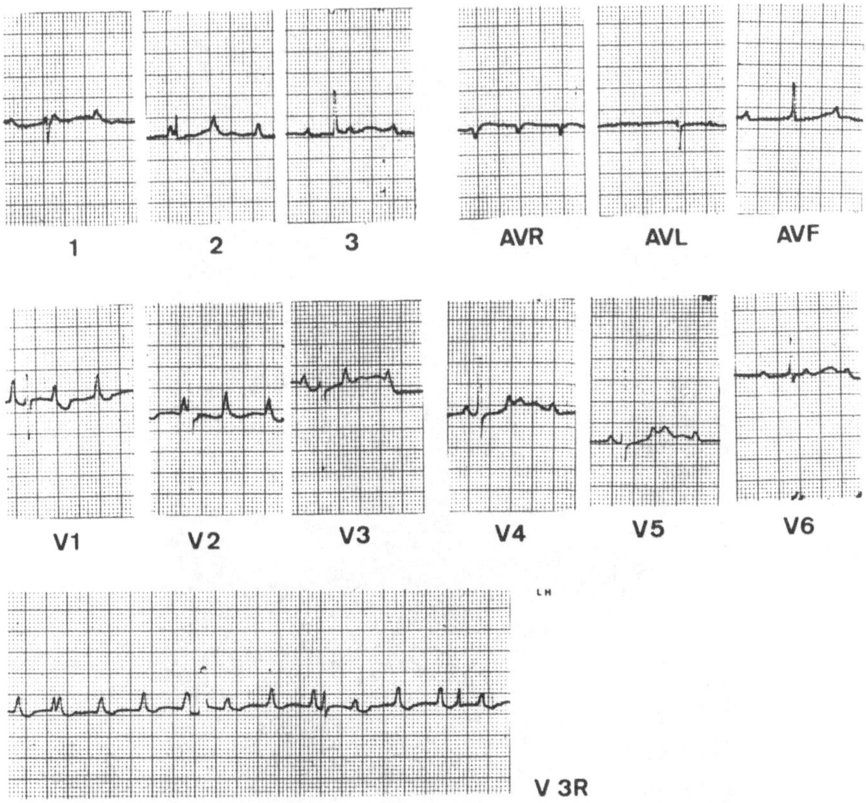

Figure 1. Electrocardiogram of patient 1. There is complete heart block with an atrial rate of 150 beats/min. and a ventricular rate of 50 beats/min. The morphology of the QRS complexes suggests a ventricular pacemaking site high in the left side of the ventricular septum.

cularis and the most proximal parts of the interventricular septum. This block was serially sectioned into 10 micron thick sections, perpendicular to the plane of the atrioventricular junction (fig. 2).

The entirety of the interatrial septum, beneath the atrial septal defect, was devoid of myocardial muscle. The inferior limbus consisted of sparse connective tissue fibers, intermingled with fatty tissue, venous channels and nerve trunks. A compact node was not identified at the anticipated site. However, small strands of cells, reminiscent of the specialized conduction system, were present within the anulus fibrosus. When traced anteriorly, these archipelagoes condensed into a well defined atrioventricular bundle. The left bundle

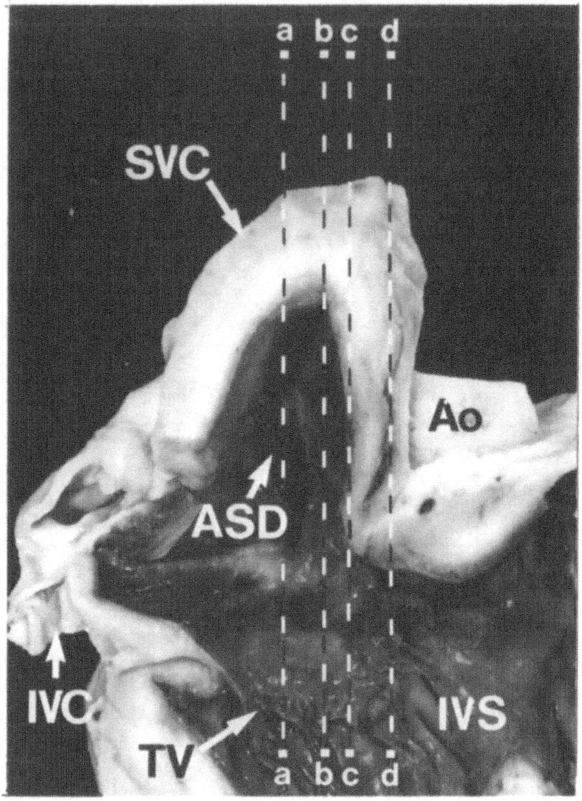

Figure 2. Photograph of the block of tissue removed for histological sectioning from Case 1. The block contains the entirety of the interatrial septum, including the ostia of the superior (SVC) and inferior venae cavae (IVC) and the coronary sinus. The atrioventricular septal junction is also included. The lines a-a through d-d indicate the plane of section, at right angles to the atrioventricular junction. Photomicrographs of these sections are shown in figure 3. Ao = aorta; TV = tricuspid valve; IVS = interventricular septum; ASD = atrial septal defect.

Figure 3. Histology of the atrioventricular junctional area of Case 1. The photomicrographs A through D have been taken at the sites a-a through d-d, as indicated in figure 2. Right-left orientation is indicated in the panels A and B. Fig. 3A shows that the inferior limbus of the interatrial septum (IAS) is not composed of myocardium but contains only fatty and fibrous tissue. At the site of the anticipated atrioventricular node, fig. 3B, this situation has not changed and the compact node cannot be identified. There is a firm anulus fibrosus (AF) separating atrial tissue from ventricular septal myocardium (IVS). Fig. 3C shows a bundle of conduction tissue (arrow) embedded within the collagen of the central fibrous body (CFB). This bundle never contacted atrial myocardium, but when traced anteriorly, fig. 3D, ran inferior to the membranous septum and gave rise to left bundle branches (LBB). A right bundle branch was not identified.

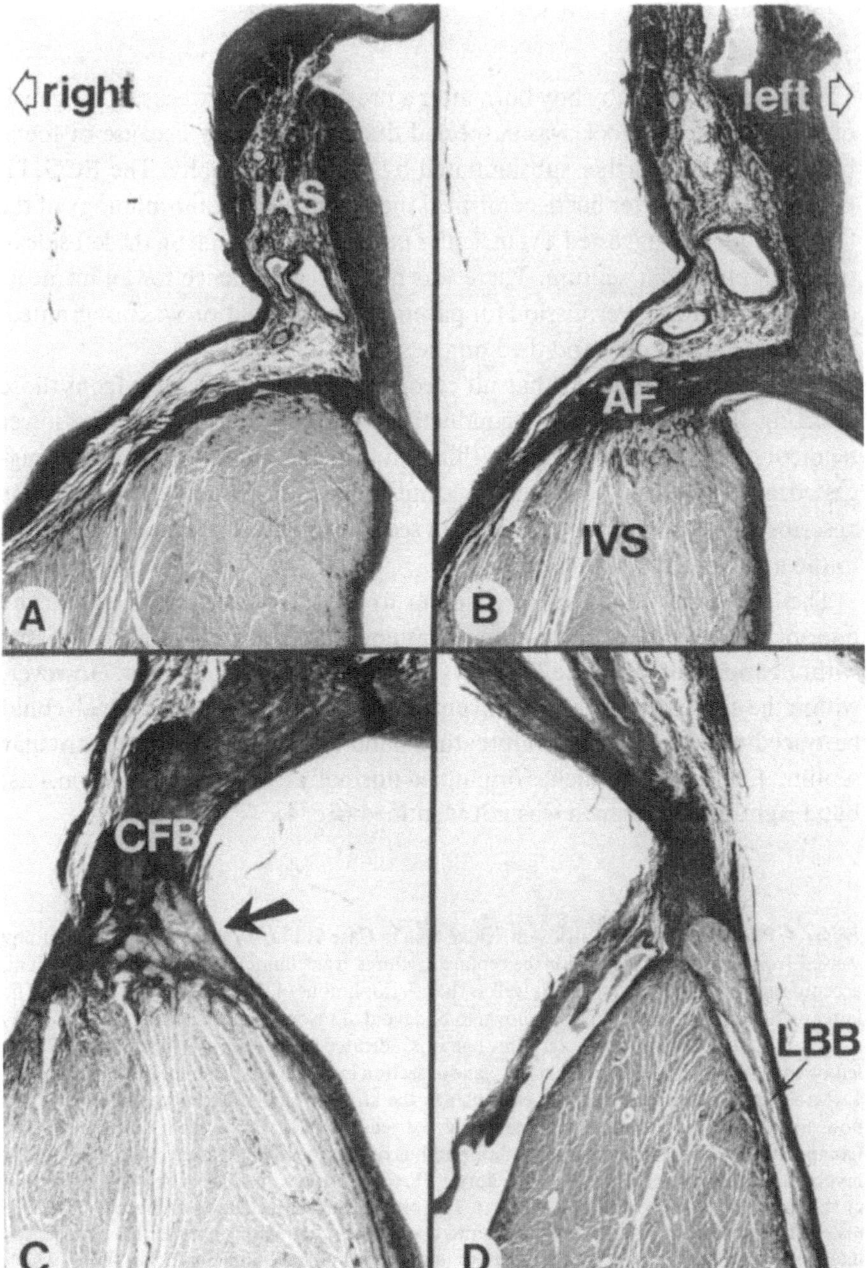
right
IAS
A
left
AF
IVS
B
CFB
C
LBB
D

branches originated normally, but a right bundle branch was not identified (fig. 3).

Patient 2

This patient was a baby boy born after a pregnancy of 42 weeks. A diagnosis of complete heart block was suspected during pregnancy because of foetal bradycardia and further substantiated by echocardiography. The ECG, taken immediately after birth, confirmed the diagnosis. The morphology of the QRS complexes suggested a ventricular pacemaker site high on the left side of the interventricular septum. There was no clinical evidence for an intracardiac malformation. Permission for pacemaker implantation was not granted; the infant deteriorated and died on the second day of life.

The autopsy confirmed that no cardiac abnormalities, apart from those affecting the atrioventricular conduction system, were present. The lower segment of the atrial septum was thin and transillumination of the area suggested absence of myocardium. A similar block of tissue was removed as described for patient 1, but the plane of sectioning in this instance was parallel to the atrioventricular junction.

The histological findings were similar to those obtained in patient 1. The inferior limbus of the atrial septum was composed entirely of fibrous tissue without appreciable muscle. There was no compact node identified. However, within the anulus fibrosus an atrioventricular bundle was present which could be traced anteriorly into a bifurcating bundle lying astride the ventricular septum. Left bundle branches originated normally from this conduction axis, but a right bundle branch was not identified (fig. 4).

Figure 4. Photographs of the atrioventricular area in Case 2. Fig. 4A shows the gross anatomy viewed from the right aspect with the septal structures transilluminated from the left atrium, accentuating the fossa ovalis (FO) as well as the inferior limbus of the atrial septum (arrow). The latter on histological sectioning was shown to be devoid of myocardium. The plane of section, as illustrated in the photomicrographs B through D is indicated by the lines b-b, through d-d. Right-left orientation as in fig. 3. Note that the plane of section in this case is different from that in Case 1. Rather than being sectioned perpendicular to the atrioventricular junction, the sections are now taken in a more or less parallel plane. TV = tricuspid valve; RV = right ventricle. Fig. 4B (compare to line b-b) shows that the inferior limbus of the interatrial septum (IAS) contains no myocardium. MV = mitral valve; Ao = aorta; TV = tricuspid valve. Fig. 4C (compare to line c-c) shows a bundle of conduction tissue (CT) which never contacted atrial myocardium, but instead first appeared embedded within fibrous tissue of the central fibrous body. PS = posterior interventricular septum. Fig. 4D (compare to line d-d) shows left bundle branches (LBB) which originated from the bundle illustrated in fig. 4C. A right bundle branch was not identified in this case.

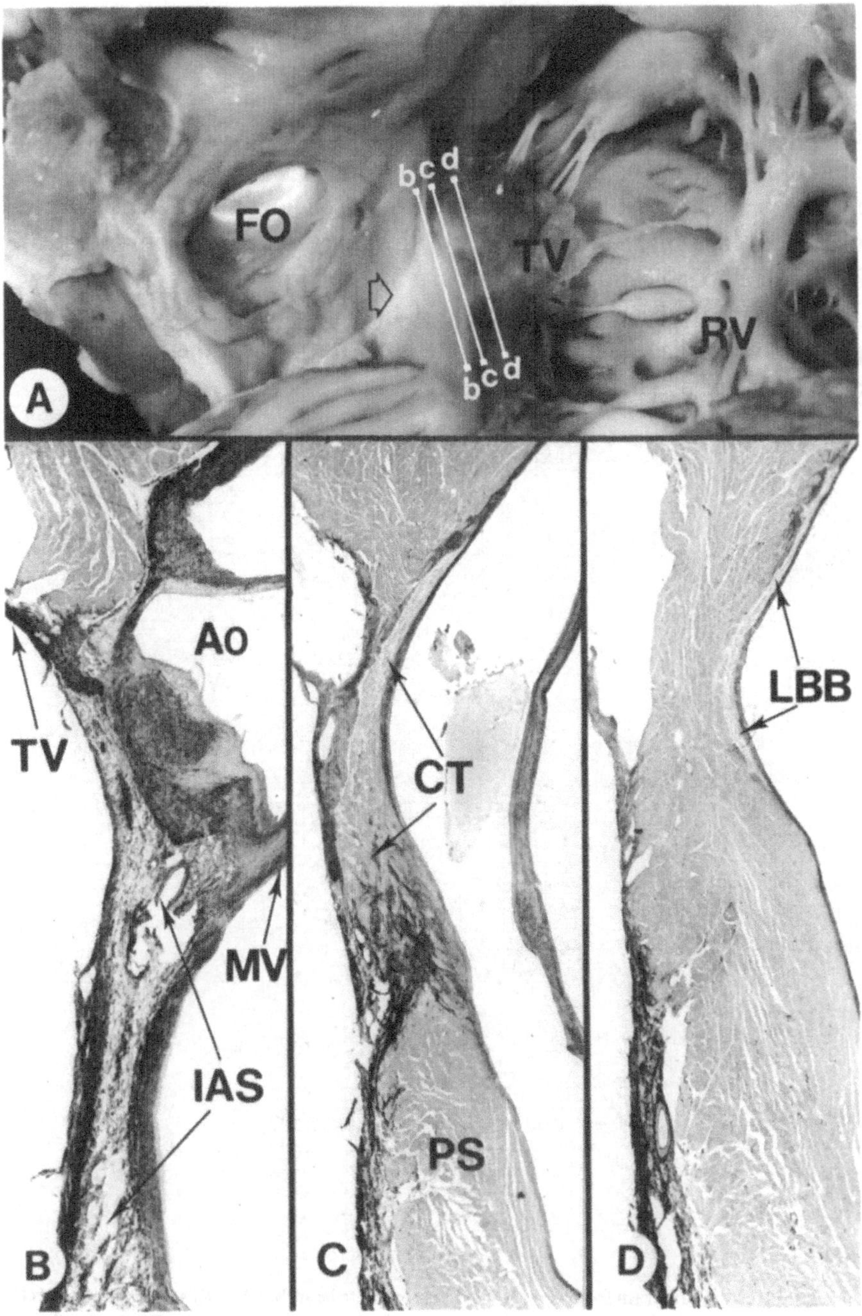
A
FO
b c d
b c d
TV
RV
B
TV
Ao
MV
IAS
C
CT
PS
D
LBB

Patient 3

This baby girl was born spontaneously after a pregnancy of 36 weeks. Foetal bradycardia had been noted during pregnancy and echocardiography had confirmed the diagnosis of congenitally complete heart block. The intra-uterine ventricular rate had been 55 beats per minute which fell to 35 beats per minute after birth. Postnatal investigations confirmed the diagnosis of congenitally complete heart block and the QRS morphology suggested a ventricular focus high on the right aspect of the interventricular septum (fig. 5). There were no indications of an intracardiac abnormality.

After birth the heart rate slowed to 30 beats per minute, accompanied by progressive cardiac failure and despite intensive medical therapy the baby died at the age of 2 days.

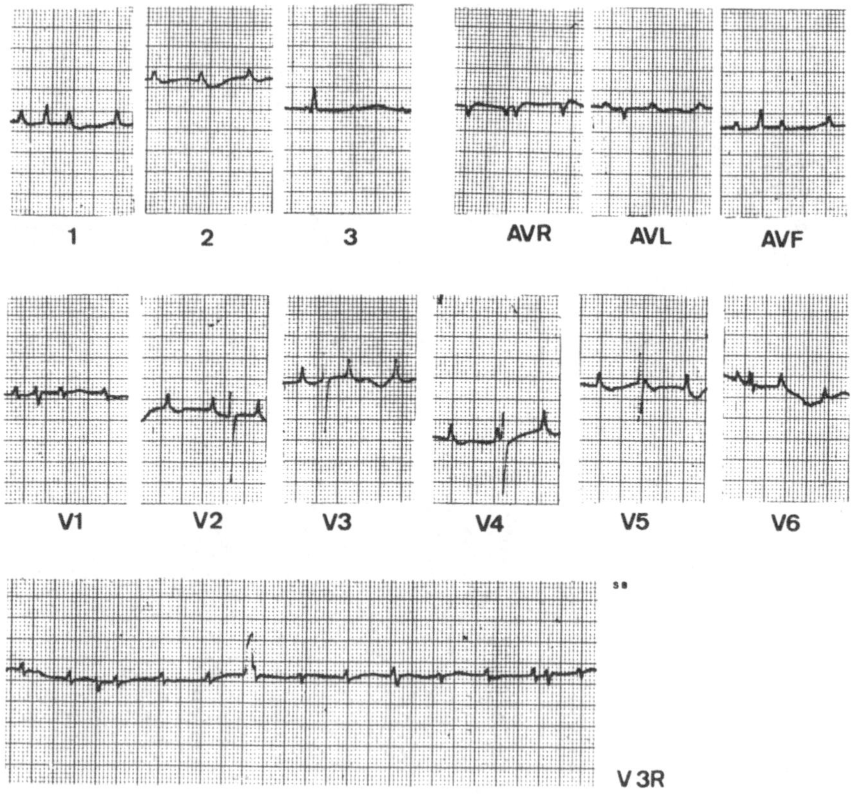

Figure 5. Electrocardiogram from Case 3. There is complete heart block with an atrial rate of 140 beats/min. and a ventricular rate of 44 beats/min. The morphology of the QRS complexes suggested a high right septal focus for the ventricular activation.

The autopsy confirmed absence of intracardiac abnormalities. The inferior limbus of the atrial septum did not show the abnormalities as noted previously. A similar block of tissue was removed for histological examination of the atrioventricular conduction system and was sectioned in the same plane as described for patient 1.

In this heart the atrioventricular node and transitional cell zone were well formed and normally situated. However, when traced anteriorly, the nodal-bundle axis faded out to disappear within the dense connective tissue of the anulus fibrosus. In a more anterior plane a ventricular conduction bundle was identified. The right and left bundle branches took origin from this bundle in a normal fashion (fig. 6).

DISCUSSION

Our observations in three hearts of patients with congenitally complete heart block further substantiate the concept that the definitive atrioventricular conduction tissues in the human heart develop from different sources.

In our first and second patients there was complete absence of the proximal parts of the atrioventricular junctional area. Both the transitional cell zone and the compact node were absent. Minute archipelagoes of specialized conduction cells, embedded within the anulus fibrosus, could be traced into a well defined bifurcating bundle positioned at the crest of the interventricular septum. With relation to concepts of development of the normal atrioventricular junctional area (7-10) one could argue that in both these instances a faulty development of the specialized atrioventricular ring tissue had occurred. However, this concept does not necessarily clarify why the transitional cell zone failed to develop. One might speculate that the development of this zone depends upon the development of the proximal part of the conduction axis. It is of interest, in this respect, that a case has as yet to be reported in literature, where transitional cell zone was absent in the presence of a normally developed compact node. All cases of congenitally complete heart block due to lack of contact between atrial myocardium and conduction tissue, thusfar reported, have shown a deficiency of the transitional cell zone accompanied by either an absent, a fragmented or a hypoplastic node, embedded within the collagen of the central fibrous body (2, 4-6, 10, 11). In the first two cases the morphology of the QRS complexes suggested a ventricular pacemaker focus localized at the left side of the ventricular septum, close to the atrioventricular junctional area. In both instances, the conduction tissue axis was found on

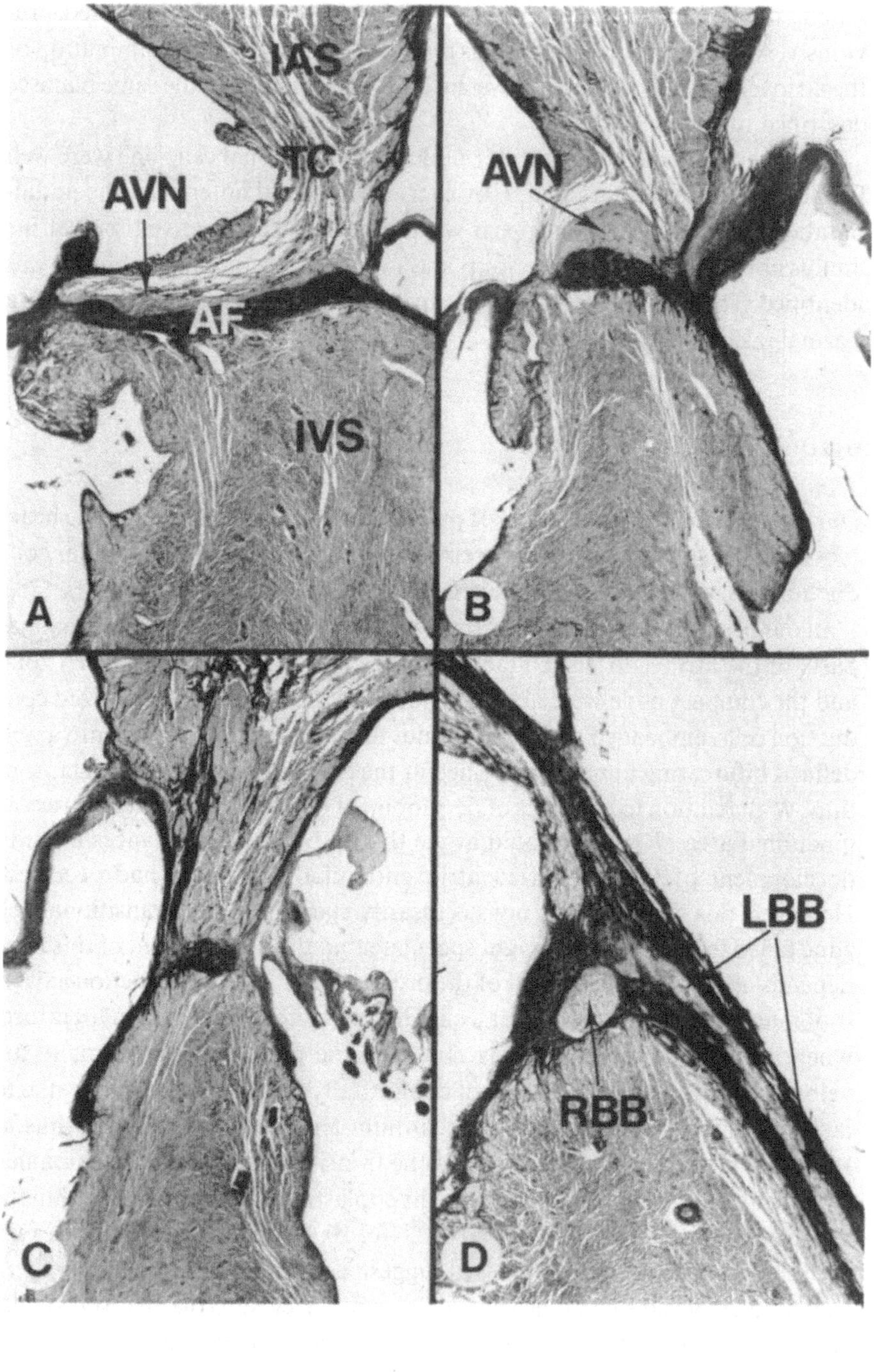
IAS
TC
AVN
AF
IVS
A
AVN
B
C
LBB
RBB
D

top of the ventricular septum with only left bundle branches present. The significance of this observation, as far as predicting the type of developmental error underlying the atrioventricular block, needs further evaluation.

Our observations in the third case differ in that a well developed proximal atrioventricular junctional area was present, albeit in complete isolation from the distal conduction axis. From the developmental scheme this can be accounted for on the basis of failure of fusion between the proximal segment, derived from the atrioventricular specialized ring tissue, and the distal segment, derived from the ventriculo-bulbar ring tissue. Failure of fusion in this instance is not due to faulty septation of the heart but probably relates to an intrinsic abnormality in the formation of the nodal-bundle conduction axis. To assume that the abnormality relates to persistence of 'sulcus tissue' at the site of fusion is speculative, but the observation fits within such a developmental concept (10).

It is our opinion that the three pathologic specimens are in accord with a concept of an *in situ* segmental development of the atrioventricular conduction system.

In summary, from a histological standpoint, congenitally complete heart block in an otherwise normal heart can be divided into cases with discontinuity between the atrium and ventricular conduction tissues and cases with nodal-bundle discontinuity, as previously suggested by Lev (1, 3-6). Whether this anatomical finding has clinical significance remains to be established.

REFERENCES

1. Lev, M., Pathogenesis of congenital atrioventricular block. *Prog. Cardiovasc. Dis.* 15, 145 (1972).
2. Carter, J. B., Blieden, I. C. and Edwards, J. E., Congenital heart block, anatomic correlations and review of the literature. *Arch. Pathol.* 98, 51 (1974).

◀ *Figure 6*. Photomicrographs of the atrioventricular junction area in Case 3. The sections have been cut at right angles to the anulus fibrosus, comparable to those illustrated in the figs. 2 and 3. Right-left orientation as in fig. 3. Fig. 6A shows the posterior aspects of the atrioventricular node (AVN) contacted by transitional cells (TC) which stream downwards from the interatrial septum (IAS). The atrioventricular node is separated from the interventricular septum (IVS) by a well formed anulus fibrosus (AF). Fig. 6B shows a more anterior plane of section with a well formed compact node (AVN) still separated from the ventricular musculature by the collagen barrier of the anulus fibrosus. When traced anteriorly, fig. 6C, the atrioventricular node did not penetrate the central fibrous body, but instead faded out and disappeared completely. However, at a more anterior level, as illustrated in fig. 6D a bundle of conduction tissue was again present from which the left (LBB) and right (RBB) bundle branches originated.

3. Lev, M., Paul, M. H. and Cassels, D. E., Complete atrioventricular block associated with atrial septal defects of the fossa ovalis (secundum) type. *Am. J. Cardiol.* 19, 266 (1967).
4. Lev, M., Silverman, J., Fitzmaurice, F. M., Paul, M. H., Cassels, D. E. and Miller, R. A., Lack of connection between the atria and the more peripheral conduction system in congenital atrioventricular block. *Am. J. Cardiol.* 27, 481 (1971).
5. Lev, M., Cuadros, H. and Paul, M. H., Interruption of the atrioventricular bundle with congenital atrioventricular block. *Circulation* 43, 703 (1971).
6. Miller, R. A., Mehta, A. B., Rodriguez-Colonel, A. and Lev, M., Congenital atrioventricular block with multiple ectopic pacemakers. *Am. J. Cardiol.* 30, 554 (1972).
7. James, T. N., Cardiac conduction system: fetal and postnatal development. *Am. J. Cardiol.* 25, 213 (1970).
8. Anderson, R. H. and Taylor, I. M., Development of atrioventricular specialized tissue in human heart. *Br. Heart J.* 34, 1205 (1972).
9. Wenink, A. C. G., Development of the human cardiac conducting system. *J. Anat.* 121, 617 (1976).
10. Anderson, R. H., Wenink, A. C. G., Losekoot, T. G. and Becker, A. E., Congenitally complete heart block. Developmental aspects. *Circulation* 56, 90 (1977).
11. Théry, C., Lekieffre, J. and Dupuis, C., Les blocs auriculoventriculaires congénitaux du nourrisson. *Arch. Mal. Coeur* 68, 1095 (1975).

6. THE CONDUCTING SYSTEM IN HEARTS WITH ATRIOVENTRICULAR CANAL MALFORMATIONS*

A. C. G. WENINK, R. H. ANDERSON AND G. THIENE

INTRODUCTION AND EMBRYOLOGIC REMARKS

Common atrioventricular canal can be present in its partial or complete forms. In the complete form, there is an atrial septal defect of the ostium primum type, a common valve whose anterior and posterior leaflets hang across the rim of the ventricular septum without contacting each other, and a ventricular septal defect in a posterior position. In other words, there is a combined atrial and ventricular septal defect with free floating common valve leaflets half way across this defect.

The partial form (or ostium primum defect) differs in only one respect: there is no ventricular septal defect. This, however, seems to be simply a matter of valvular attachment. In ostium primum hearts, the rim of the ventricular septum is still too low, but it provides attachment for the valve leaflets, either directly, or by means of a ridge of fibrous tissue. Seen from the left, the common valve assumes the appearance of a split septal leaflet of the mitral valve. Since the development of the atrioventricular valves is an extremely late manifestation in cardiac development, the mode of attachment or non-attachment of the common valve leaflets is thought to be secondary to the underlying disorder. This disorder in partial and complete forms is absent or incomplete septation of the atrioventricular canal. The result is always a common atrioventricular fibrous anulus.

Since we think that septation of the atrioventricular canal is a primary event which enables the endocardial cushions to fuse, we feel that the term endocardial cushion defect (1, 2, 3) is not advisable, and the name persistent (common) atrioventricular canal (4, 5, 6) should be preferred. Indeed, the term is also applicable to ostium primum hearts.

The role of the endocardial cushions in the formation of the fibrous anuli is minimal. Much more weight is ascribed to the role of the external sulcus tissue

* Part of this study was supported by a grant from the Netherlands Heart Foundation.

(7, 8). Anterior and posterior invagination of the atrioventricular canal leads to a continuity of fibrous tissue through the cavity of the heart. Most of the central fibrous body is formed from sulcus tissue. Similarly, the tendon of Todaro is principally an external structure. This tendon, initially called the tendon of the Eustachian valve (9, 10) was termed the tendon of Todaro by Scaffidi (11) and has been so called since (12, 13).

Invagination of the sinus venosus into the right part of the atrium brings sulcus tissue inwards. The right venous valve contains fibrous tissue which becomes continuous with the fibrous tissue invaginated from the anterior side. Todaro (9) described this tissue as a tendon which continued from the central fibrous body into the posterior epicardium. Fibrous tissue has been observed in the Eustachian valve from embryonic stages on (10). In animals lacking a Eustachian valve a fibrous strand in the posterior atrial wall has been described as the homologue of Todaro's tendon (11). Todaro's tendon is an important point of reference for the localization of the atrioventricular node in the normal heart (see Anderson and Becker, this book, pp. 28-30).

Septation of the atrioventricular canal has direct effects upon atrium and ventricle. Therefore, deficient atrioventricular septation is linked to deficient septation of the atrium and of the ventricle. This explains the deficiency of the posterior portion of the ventricular septum in both the partial and complete forms of the atrioventricular canal malformation, which has previously been noted (14).

DISPOSITION OF THE CONDUCTING SYSTEM

The above considerations are necessary to understand the disposition of the conducting system in this malformation. There is again no notable difference between partial and complete forms.

The, frequently hypoplastic, atrioventricular node has an abnormally posterior position. Its relationship to the fibrous tissues of sinus septum and atrioventricular anulus is comparable to the normal. As would be expected, however, Todaro's tendon is abnormal (fig. 1). Its anterior portion arises from the anterior remnant of the central fibrous body and courses posteriorly through the rim of the deficient atrial septum. Near the coronary sinus, which itself is displaced posteriorly, it regains relationships with the fibrous anulus reminiscent of the normal.

The penetrating bundle, too, is displaced posteriorly. It lies on the rim of the ventricular septum and its exact course depends on the degree of

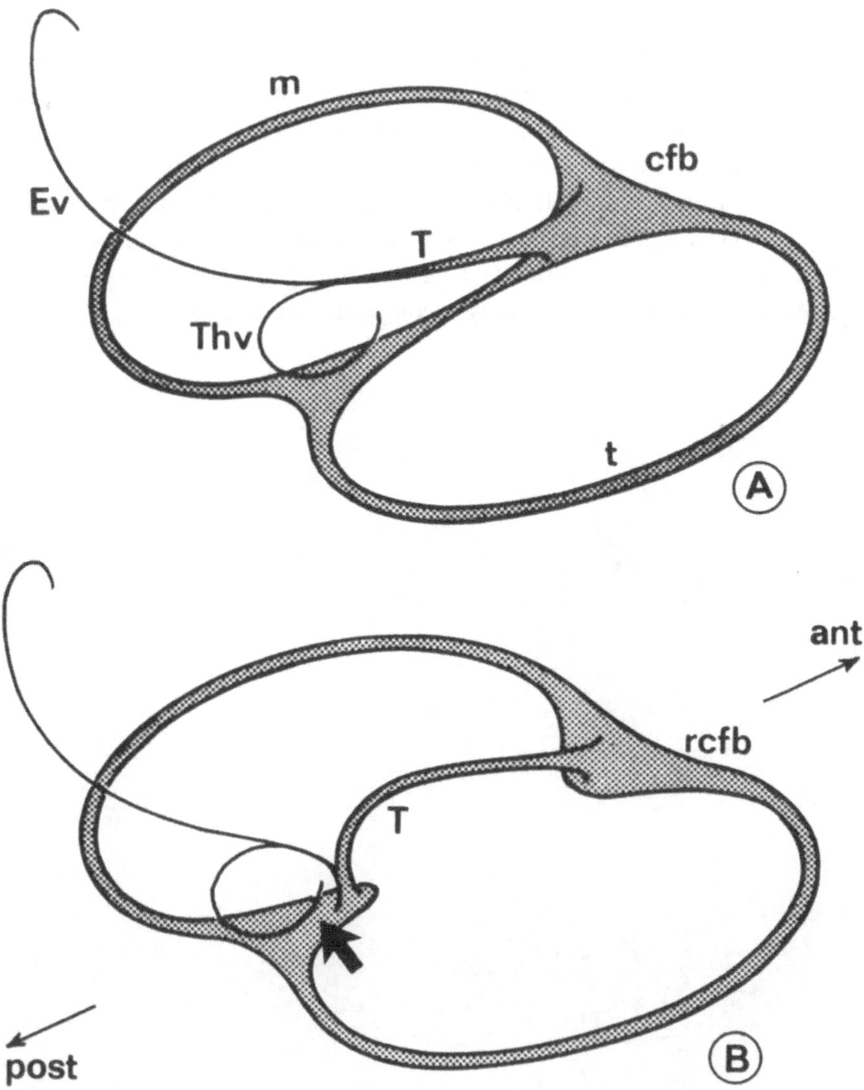

Figure 1. Diagram to show the differences of the fibrous heart skeletons in the normal heart (A) and in common atrioventricular canal (B). In the latter, the central fibrous body (cfb) is greatly deficient. The course of Todaro's tendon (T) is abnormal: it lies in the free rim of the atrial septum. The position of the atrioventricular node is far posterior, behind the continuity of Todaro's tendon and the posterior portion of the fibrous anulus (arrow). Ev: rim of Eustachian valve; Thv: rim of Thebesian valve; m: mitral anulus; t: tricuspid anulus; rcfb: remnant of central fibrous body.

deficiency of the ventricular septum. In complete forms, the bundle will be bare on the septum. In the partial form, however, it is covered by the fibrous tissue, which connects the malformed valve leaflets to the septum. Microscopically, this tissue may have the appearance of a membranous septum (fig. 2). Additionally, the penetrating bundle has a longer course before reaching the bifurcation. This, again is at an abnormally posterior site.

As a consequence, the left bundle branch, too, originates more posteriorly than normal. Its posterior fibres are therefore abnormally close to the posterior wall of the left ventricle. This is felt to explain the left superior axis deviation which almost invariably accompanies the anomaly.

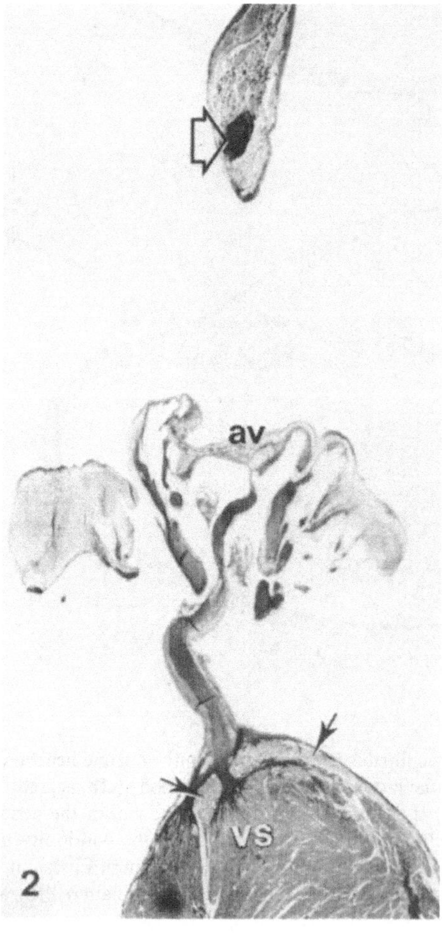

Figure 2. Frontal section of a case of common atrioventricular canal (complete form). Note the tendon of Todaro (open arrow) in the rim of the atrial septum. Between the common valve (av) and the ventricular septum (vs) fibrous tissue is present which closely resembles a normal membranous septum. Arrows: right and left bundle branches.

DISCUSSION

In general, our anatomic findings are in keeping with those obtained by Lev (4), Feldt et al. (15) and Wolff and Alley (16), and are in agreement with the embryologic considerations given above.

Lack of atrioventricular septation is the cause of the common atrioventricular anulus. At the same time, not only the fibrous tissues remain at more or less embryonic sites, but the same holds for the specialized myocardium in the atrioventricular transition. On the one hand, the posterior indentation of the atrioventricular ring forming the central part of the node, has kept a relative posterior position. On the other hand, the anterior indentation has remained anterior and has not been able to contribute to the node (fig. 3), thus frequently producing a hypoplastic node in a posterior position. As stated, this node has nearly normal relations with the posterior fibrous tissues, but its great distance to the anterior remnant of the central fibrous body is abnormal. Alternatively, the anterior portion of the tendon of Todaro has normal relations to this remnant of the central fibrous body. In one case, the

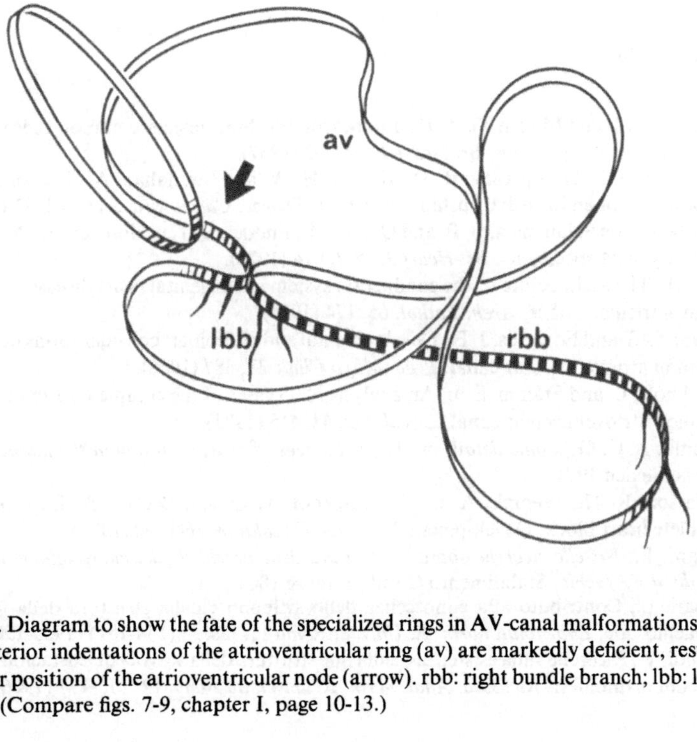

Figure 3. Diagram to show the fate of the specialized rings in AV-canal malformations. Anterior and posterior indentations of the atrioventricular ring (av) are markedly deficient, resulting in a posterior position of the atrioventricular node (arrow). rbb: right bundle branch; lbb: left bundle branch. (Compare figs. 7-9, chapter I, page 10-13.)

fibrous tissues at this site were in addition seen to be normally related to the specialized myocardium. The anterior part of the atrioventricular specialized ring which, of course, had not been able to contribute to the node could be distinguished wedged between Todaro's tendon and the remnant of the central fibrous body. Here, prolonged presence of specialized myocardium provides additional arguments for the explanation of this malformation.

The deficient septation of the atrioventricular canal is closely linked to the deficient development of the posterior part of the ventricular septum. It is felt, that the posterior part of the septum arises by the very developmental process which produces partitioning of the atrioventricular canal. This portion is essentially too low in common atrioventricular canals. Characteristic for this part of the septum is that it carries the bundle, and an explanation is thus given for the aberrant course of the latter.

The contact between atrioventricular and bulboventricular rings is at the boundary between the posterior septal portion and the rest of the septum. As a consequence of the hypoplasia of the posterior portion, the bifurcation, too, lies more posteriorly than normal (fig. 3). The posterior fibres of the left bundle branch are especially subject to such a displacement.

REFERENCES

1. Campbell, M. and Missen, G. A. K., Endocardial cushion defects: common atrioventricular canal and ostium primum. *Br. Heart J.* 19, 403 (1957).
2. Van Mierop, L. H. S., Alley, R. D., Kausel, H. W. and Stranahan, A., The anatomy and embryology of endocardial cushion defects. *J. Thorac. Cardiovasc. Surg.* 43, 71 (1962).
3. Ugarte, M., de Salamanca, F. E. and Quero, M., Endocardial cushion defects. An anatomical study of 54 specimens. *Br. Heart J.* 38-7, 674 (1976).
4. Lev, M., The architecture of the conduction system in congenital heart disease. I. Common atrioventricular orifice. *Arch. Pathol.* 65, 174 (1958).
5. Wakai, C. S. and Edwards, J. E., Developmental and pathologic considerations in persistent common atrioventricular canal. *Proc. Mayo Clinic* 31, 487 (1956).
6. Tenckhoff, L. and Stamm, S. J., An analysis of 35 cases of the complete form of persistent common atrioventricular canal. *Circulation* 48, 416 (1973).
7. Wenink, A. C. G., *Some details on the final stages of heart septation in the human embryo.* Thesis, Leiden 1971.
8. Anderson, R. H., Wenink, A. C. G., Losekoot, T. G. and Becker, A. E., Congenitally complete heart block. Developmental aspects. *Circulation* 56-1, 90 (1977).
9. Todaro, F., *Novelle ricerche sopra la struttura delle orechielle del cuore umano e sopra la valvola di Eustachio.* Stabilimento Civelli, Firenze 1865.
10. Versari, L., Contributo alla conoscenza dello sviluppo e della struttura della valvola di Eustachio. *Ric. Lab. Anat. norm. R. Univ. di Roma* 11, fasc. 3 (154-181) (1905-1906).
11. Scaffidi, V., Ricerche sulla esistenza e sulla fine struttura della valvola di Eustachio nel cuore di alcuni mammiferi. *Ric. Lab. Anat. norm. R. università Roma* 12: 178-197 (1906-1907).

12. Wolner, E., Die Todarosche Sehne. *Z. Anat. Entw. gesch.* 124, 114 (1965).
13. Becker, A. E. and Anderson, R. H., Morphology of the human atrioventricular junctional area. In: Wellens, Lie and Janse (ed.) *The conduction system of the heart. Structure, function and clinical implications.* H. E. Stenfert Kroese, B.V., Leiden (1976).
14. Goor, D., Lillehei, C. W. and Edwards, J. E., Further observations on the pathology of atrioventricular canal malformation. *Arch. Surg.* 97, 954 (1968).
15. Feldt, R. H., DuShane, J. W. and Titus, J. L., The atrioventricular conduction system in persistent common atrioventricular canal defect: correlations with electrocardiogram. *Circulation* 42, 437 (1970).
16. Wolff, G. S. and Alley, R. D., Intraoperative identification of the conduction system in repair of endocardial cushion defect. *Ann. Thorac. Surg.* 23-1, 39 (1977).

7. CONDUCTING TISSUE IN THE UNIVENTRICULAR HEART*

R. H. ANDERSON, J. L. WILKINSON AND A. E. BECKER

INTRODUCTION

Before describing conducting tissue in the univentricular heart, it is necessary to define a univentricular heart. This is dependant upon giving a precise definition of ventricles as opposed to rudimentary chambers. Much of the controversy which surrounds univentricular hearts derives from the fact that most authorities consider a normal ventricle as possessing only two portions, namely sinus and conus (1, 2). This system is admirable when chambers receive atrioventricular valves, but problems arise when a given chamber does not receive an atrioventricular valve. In the setting of 'single ventricle with outlet chamber', such chambers are tacitly assumed *not* to be ventricles (1, 2). However, in the setting of 'tricuspid atresia', similar chambers are described as ventricles merely because of the larger size of their trabeculated component (3). Such a Procrustean approach is unnecessary if normal ventricles are considered as possessing *three* components, as proposed by Goor and his colleagues (4, 5). These components are the inlet portion related to an atrioventricular valve, be that valve perforate or imperforate, the trabecular portion which conveys 'rightness' or 'leftness' on a chamber and the outlet portion or infundibulum which supports an arterial valve (fig. 1). Using this approach, the normal ventricular septum can similarly be considered to possess three muscular portions, the inlet septum, the trabecular septum and the infundibular septum.

DEFINITIONS OF VENTRICLES AND RUDIMENTARY CHAMBERS

Within the definition given above, to be considered as a ventricle a chamber *must* possess an inlet portion. When this inlet portion straddles a septum, be it

* Supported by a grant from the British Heart Foundation.

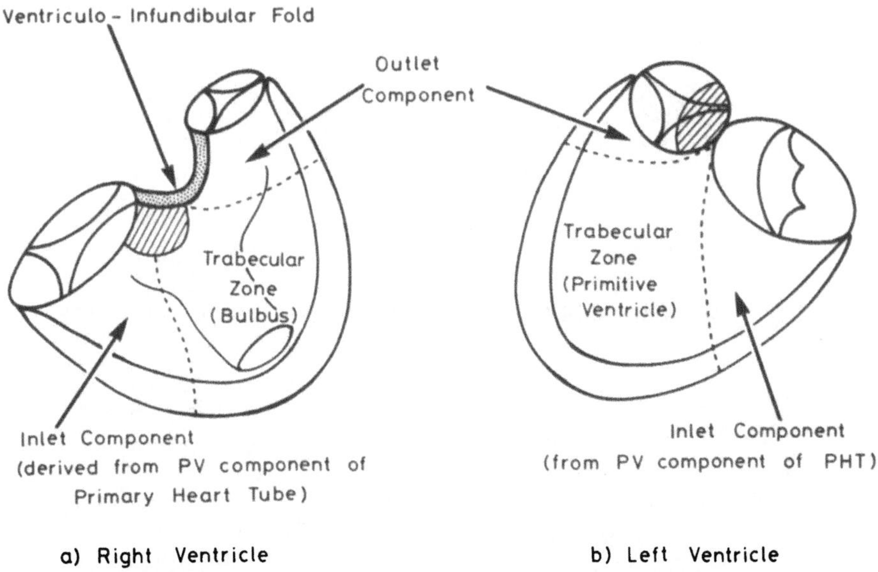

Figure 1. Diagram illustrating the developmental and morphological components of the normal right and left ventricles.

an inlet or trabecular septum, the straddling inlet portion is assigned to the chamber receiving greater than half the circumference of its atrioventricular valve. All chambers which do not possess more than half an inlet portion are described as rudimentary chambers.

Univentricular hearts can then be defined as all hearts which possess a rudimentary chamber, together with all hearts with a single chamber in their ventricular mass.

TYPES OF UNIVENTRICULAR HEART

There are three forms of ventricular morphology which produce a univentricular heart (fig. 2). They are firstly *univentricular hearts of left ventricular type with rudimentary chamber*, secondly *univentricular hearts of right ventricle type with rudimentary chamber* and thirdly *univentricular hearts without rudimentary chambers* (table 1). Huge ventricular septal defects can also produce the appearance of a univentricular heart, but since both trabecular zones can be recognized within the main chamber, they are not defined as such. Nonetheless, they will be considered from the standpoint of their con-

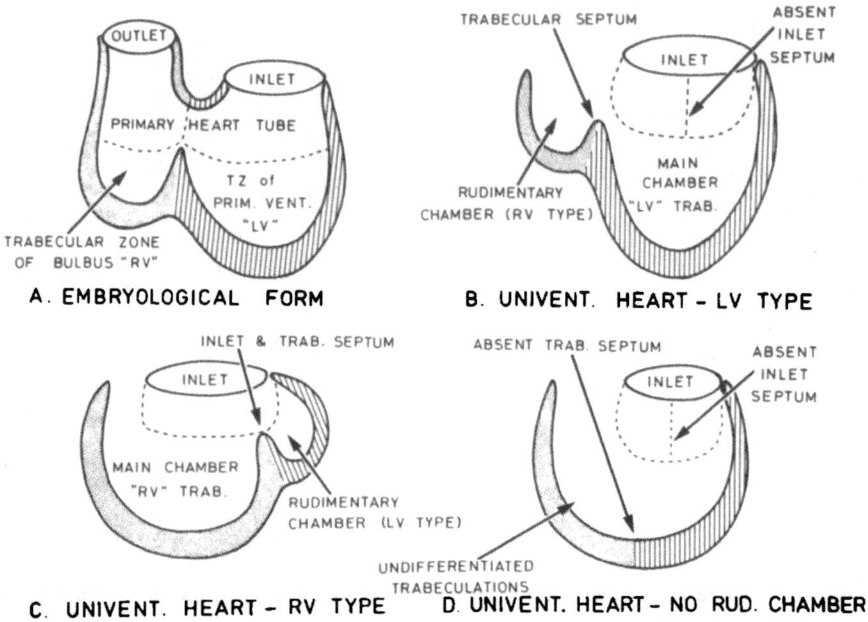

Figure 2. Diagram illustrating the possible types of univentricular heart, their embryological derivation and their septal components, if present. (TZ - trabecular zone; RV - right ventricle; LV - left ventricle).

Table 1. Classification of the Univentricular Heart.

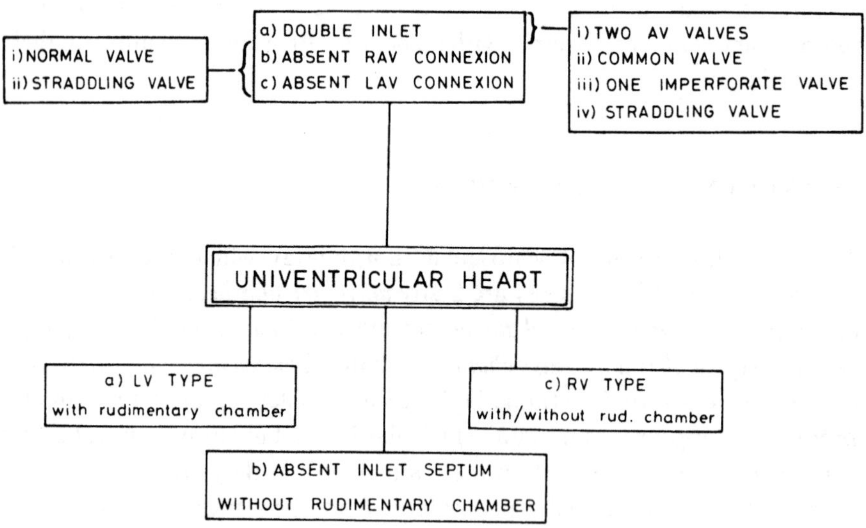

ducting tissue. The disposition of the conducting tissues in these hearts is best understood if brief consideration is first given to the morphogenesis of the anomalous ventricular masses.

MORPHOGENESIS OF UNIVENTRICULAR HEART OF LEFT VENTRICULAR TYPE WITH RUDIMENTARY CHAMBER

The hallmark of this variety is absence of the inlet portion of the ventricular septum, defined as that part of the ventricular septum which normally extends to the crux of the heart (fig. 3). The septum present is the trabecular septum (that septum which separates the trabecular zones) and always extends to the acute margin of the atrioventricular junction (fig. 3). The rudimentary chamber has right ventricular characteristics since it possesses the trabecular component derived from the bulbus. In contrast, the main chamber has left ven-

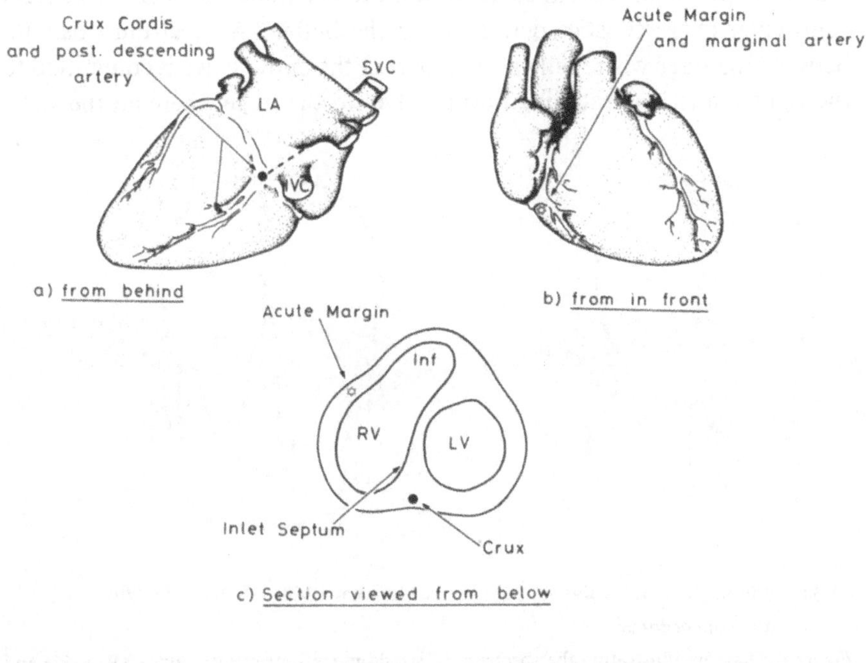

Figure 3. Diagram illustrating the position of the crux of the heart and the acute margin of the atrioventricular junction. (LA - left atrium; IVC, SVC - inferor and superior vena cava; Inf. - infundibulum; RV - right ventricle; LV - left ventricle).

tricular characteristics since it possesses the trabecular component of the primitive ventricle. Nonetheless, the main chamber is *not* a left ventricle, since it possesses both right atrial and left atrial portions of inlet myocardium derived from the primitive ventricular component of the primary heart tube. It does *not* possess 'right ventricular' myocardium, since the trabecular zone of 'right characteristics' is part of the rudimentary chamber.

MORPHOGENESIS OF UNIVENTRICULAR HEART OF RIGHT VENTRICULAR TYPE WITH RUDIMENTARY CHAMBER

In normal development, the inlet portion of the right ventricle derived from the primitive ventricular component of the primary heart tube is transferred from the primitive ventricle to the bulbus, the inlet septum being formed between the right and left inlet portions. Evidence from malformed hearts (6) indicates that, with anomalous development, the inlet portion of the definitive left ventricle, again derived from the primary heart tube, can also be transferred across the inlet septum so as to drain to the trabecular zone with right ventricular characteristics derived from the bulbus. A spectrum exists (6) between the stage where only a small part of the mitral valve is committed to the right ventricle (straddling mitral valve) to the stage where all the valve

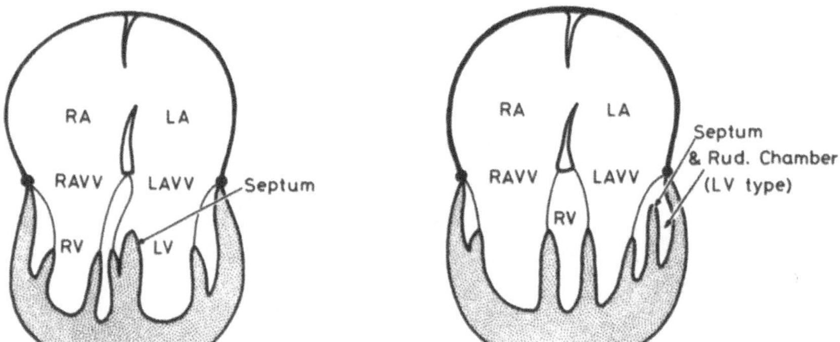

a) Straddling left AV valve — AV concordance

b) Univentricular Heart — RV type

Figure 4. Diagram illustrating the spectrum of straddling left atrioventricular (AV) valve and univentricular heart of right ventricular (RV) type dependant upon the degree of commitment of the left AV orifice. (RAVV, LAVV - right and left AV valves; RA - right atrium; other abbreviations as before).

drains to the right ventricle (fig. 4). In the latter situation the trabecular portion of the left ventricle, derived from the embryological primitive ventricle, ceases to have an inlet, and therefore becomes a rudimentary chamber of left ventricular type. Usually, such hearts have rudimentary chambers of left ventricular type, even if only slit-like cavities. However, Van Praagh et al. (1) described hearts in which the right ventricle existed in isolation, and we have seen examples of this type. It is likely that in these hearts the rudimentary chamber was completely obliterated during development. The important feature of the univentricular heart of right ventricular type is that it possesses an inlet septum, in contrast to univentricular hearts of left ventricular type where this septum is absent.

MORPHOGENESIS OF UNIVENTRICULAR HEART WITHOUT RUDIMENTARY CHAMBER

The trabecular zones of the primitive ventricle and bulbus are formed by outpouching from the original primary heart tube. Should these separate outpouchings not occur, then separate trabecular zones would not be produced, and the trabecular septum would not be formed. Our observations of univentricular hearts without rudimentary chambers are consistent with the concept that there has been failure of formation of trabecular zones, together with failure of formation of the inlet septum. Thus, as with univentricular hearts of left ventricular type, the unseptated inlets drain into the ventricular chamber, but because of failure of formation of the trabecular septum, this chamber has undifferentiated apical myocardium which has coarse trabeculations. Usually it is only the outlet portions of the heart which have septated, so that a well-formed infundibular septum is present. It is frequently difficult to differentiate these hearts from univentricular hearts of right ventricular type with small rudimentary chambers, but the distinction is important because an inlet septum is present in the latter hearts.

ATRIOVENTRICULAR CONNEXIONS IN THE UNIVENTRICULAR HEART

Within the definitions presently employed, it is important to realize that univentricular hearts can exist with the atrioventricular connexions of both double inlet ventricle (fig. 5a) or absence of one atrioventricular connexion (fig. 5b and c). In the latter condition, only a single valve connects one atrium

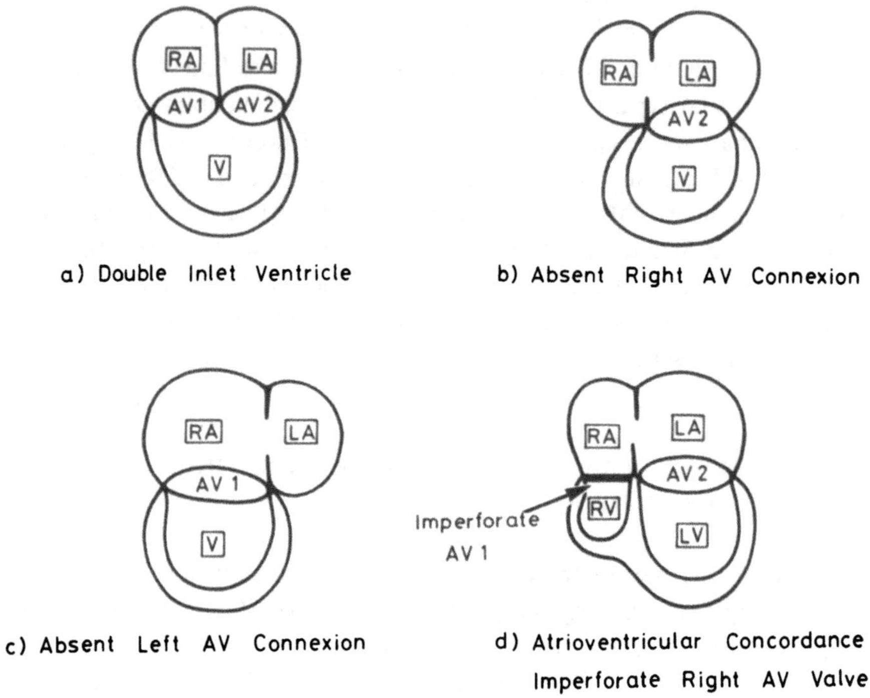

Figure 5. Diagram illustrating the modes of connexion possible in the univentricular heart (a-c) contrasted to atrioventricular concordance with an imperforate atrioventricular valve (d). (V - ventricle, morphology unspecified; AV - atrioventricular valves; other abbreviations as before).

to the ventricular mass. The other atrium is not in communication with either the main chamber or a rudimentary chamber. Such hearts comprise the majority of hearts with 'tricuspid atresia' and a minority of hearts with 'mitral atresia'. Should an imperforate membrane representing an atretic valve be additionally committed to the main chamber, then the heart is categorized as double inlet ventricle with an imperforate valve. Such a heart would be univentricular. However, should an imperforate membrane separate the blind ending atrium from the *other* chamber in the ventricular mass, then such a chamber will have an inlet portion and will *not* be a univentricular heart (fig. 5d). It is important to emphasize that double inlet or absence of the right or left atrioventricular connexion can exist with any of the ventricular morphologies producing a univentricular heart (table 1).

EMBRYOLOGY OF CONDUCTING TISSUE PERTINENT TO THE UNIVENTRICULAR HEART

It is now well established (7, 8) that the atrioventricular node develops from a complete ring of atrioventricular specialized tissue which exists in the fetal heart. This ring is usually expanded at the acute margin of the developing right ventricle. The ventricular conducting tissues develop astride the trabecular septum, possibly from a ventriculo-bulbar ring of conducting tissue (8). In the normal heart, the atrioventricular node is connected to the ventricular conducting tissues by the atrioventricular bundle, formed on the inlet portion of the septum (fig. 6a). Should the inlet septum be absent, then the normally situated node will be unable to make contact with the ventricular specialized tissues. Thus in the circumstances of primitive ventricle, the normal node will not effect atrioventricular connexions. However, because of the anterior position of the trabecular septum, its right margin is directly beneath the expansion of the atrioventricular ring tissue. In our experience, this anterior expansion then becomes the connecting atrioventricular node, and joins up with the ventricular conducting tissues (fig. 6b). Thus, the key to the disposition of conducting tissue in the univentricular heart is the presence or absence of the inlet portion of the interventricular septum.

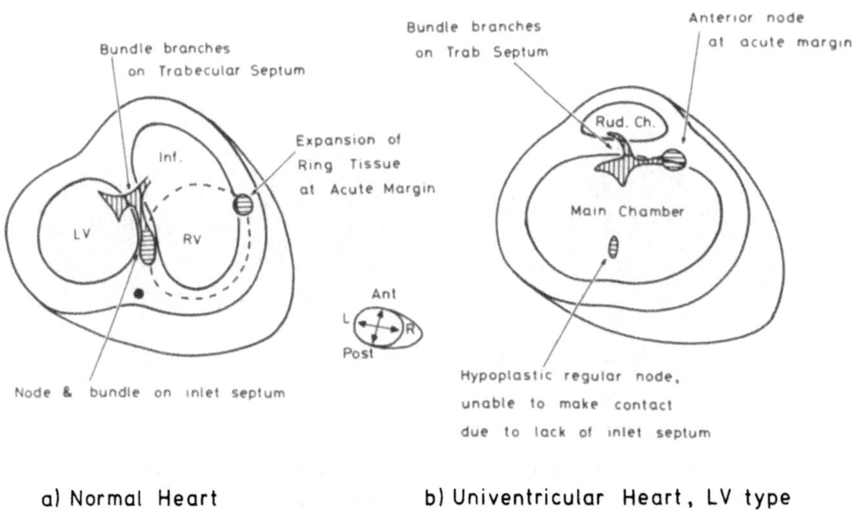

Figure 6. Diagram illustrating the disposition of conducting tissue in the normal heart as compared to that in a univentricular heart of left ventricular type.

CONDUCTING TISSUE IN UNIVENTRICULAR HEARTS

a) of Left Ventricular Type

All the univentricular hearts of left ventricular type we have studied (9) with the exception of those with absence of the right atrioventricular connexion and one other heart (vide infra) have possessed anterior atrioventricular nodes and bundles. This is because of the absence of the inlet portion of the interventricular septum. In all these hearts the posterior node was normally formed in the base of the atrial septum, but was hypoplastic since it was unable to make contact with the ventricular conducting tissues (fig. 6b). The precise course of the conducting tissue is dependant upon the position of the trabecular septum, this in itself being dependant upon the position of the rudimentary chamber. With double inlet univentricular heart of left ventricular type and left sided outlet chamber which supports an aorta, the trabecular septum is some distance from the acute margin of the right atrioventricular orifice (fig. 7a). In these circumstances, the atrioventricular bundle penetrates from the node at the acute margin, but then runs an exten-

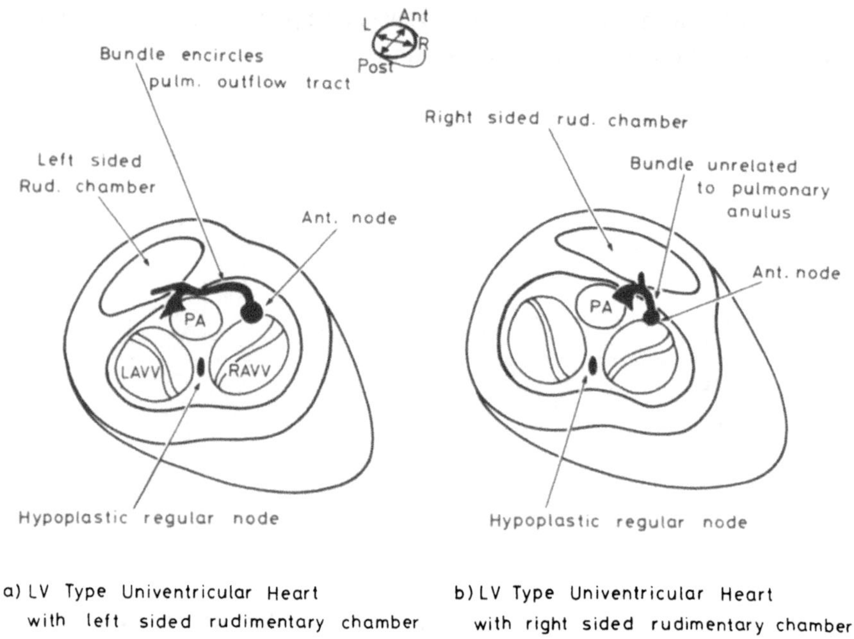

Figure 7. Diagram illustrating the course of conducting tissue in the univentricular heart of left ventricular type with left sided rudimentary chamber as opposed to the heart with right sided rudimentary chamber.

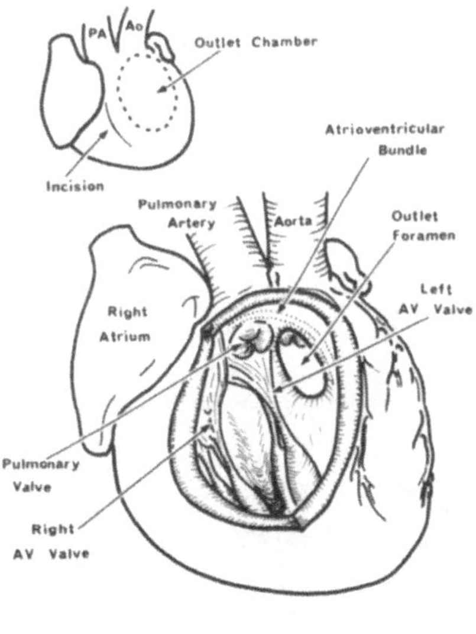

Fig. 8

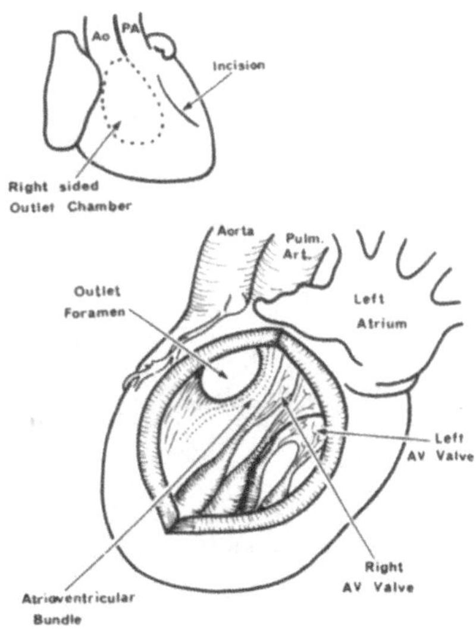

Fig. 9

Figure 8. Diagram illustrating an artist's impression of the conducting tissue disposition in univentricular heart of left ventricular type with left sided rudimentary chamber as viewed through an incision in the right side of the main chamber.

Figure 9. Diagram illustrating an artist's impression of the conducting tissue in univentricular heart of left ventricular type with right sided rudimentary chamber, as viewed through an incision in the left side of the main chamber.

sive course *anterior* to the pulmonary orifice (in the presence of ventricular-arterial discordance) before descending onto the anterior margin of the trabecular septum (fig. 8). When viewed from an incision in the right side of the main chamber the bundle runs above the pulmonary valve ring, and descends over the outlet foramen. This position is preserved in the presence of either straddling of the left atrioventricular valve or absence of the left atrioventricular connexion. When the outlet chamber supporting an aorta is right sided, then the orientation of the trabecular septum is different (fig. 7). Its posterior margin is directly beneath the acute margin of the right atrioventricular orifice, and the penetrating bundle is able to descend onto the septum without encircling the pulmonary outflow tract from the main chamber (fig. 9). The bundle therefore, unlike the situation with left sided outlet chamber, is not directly related to the pulmonary outflow tract (Compare figures 7a and b).

The disposition of conducting tissue could well be different when the outlet chamber supports the pulmonary artery (ventriculo-arterial concordance –

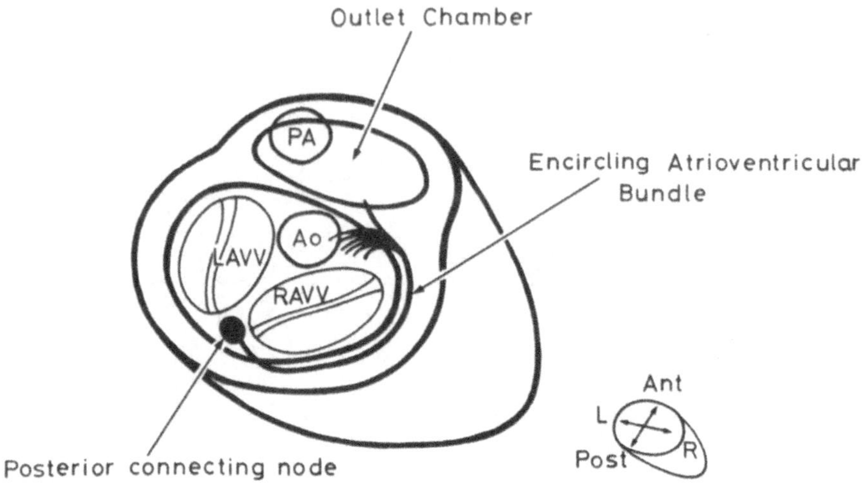

Figure 10. Diagram illustrating the unusual course of conducting tissue in a single case we have studied of univentricular heart of left ventricular type with right sided rudimentary chamber and ventriculo-arterial concordance (the so-called 'Holmes Heart'). This case may not be representative, but is the only heart of this type we have studied thus far. Abbreviations as before.

so-called 'Holmes Heart'). In the single heart we have studied of this type, the normal posterior node gave rise to a penetrating bundle, but the bundle completely encircled the right atrioventricular orifice before descending onto the posterior margin of the trabecular septum (fig. 10). In contrast, in a further heart with ventriculo-arterial concordance but a straddling right atrioventricular node, the connecting node was lateral and the bundle descended directly onto the posterior margin of the trabecular septum (fig. 11).

In hearts we have studied with univentricular heart of left ventricular type and absent right atrioventricular connexion ('Tricuspid Atresia'), the anatomy is slightly different. The right atrioventricular orifice is absent, but the connecting atrioventricular node is normally related to the landmarks of the triangle of Koch. However, the course of the penetrating bundle and its relationship to the trabecular septum are comparable with that found in double inlet ventricle of left ventricular type. This is exemplified when the course is compared with that found in examples of hypoplastic right ventricle with imperforate tricuspid valve (Compare Figures 12a and b).

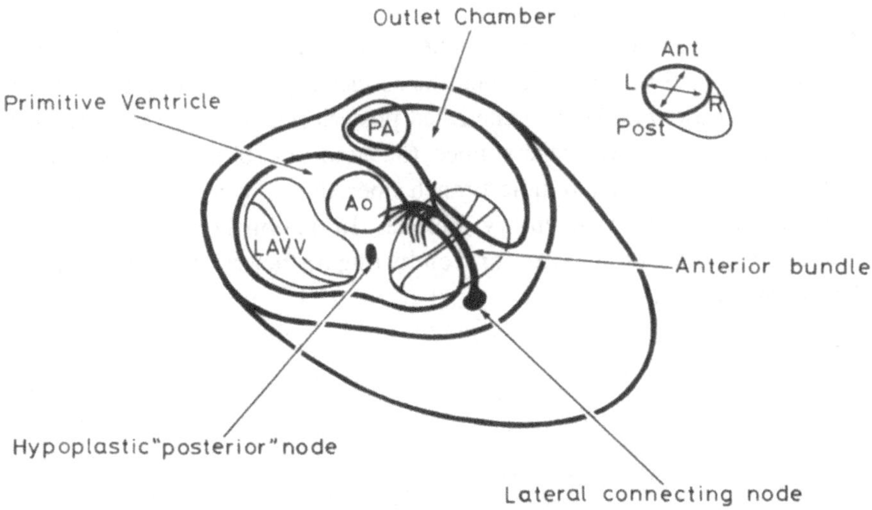

Figure 11. Diagram illustrating the disposition of conducting tissue in a single case we have studied of univentricular heart of left ventricular type, with right sided rudimentary chamber and straddling right atrioventricular valve. Although the connecting node was lateral, it was also *posterior* to the regular node.

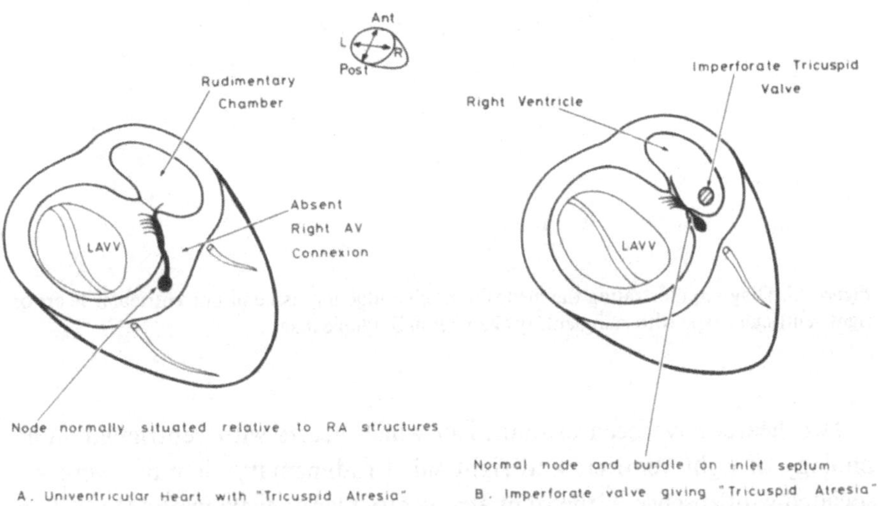

Figure 12. Diagram illustrating the differences which exist between absent right AV connexion with univentricular heart of left ventricular type ('tricuspid atresia') and atrioventricular concordance with imperforate tricuspid valve. In the former, the septum is a trabecular septum. There is an extensive bundle connecting this septum to a regular node normally located in the blind-ending right atrium. In contrast, in the latter form the bundle is normally situated on the inlet septum.

b) of Right Ventricular Type

All the hearts we have thus far examined have possessed rudimentary chambers. In the hearts with double inlet, the connecting node has been normally situated, and the bundle has penetrated posteriorly, running onto the inlet septum (fig. 13). In three hearts studied, the bundle has bifurcated on the inlet septum, and typical left bundle branch fibers have been identified on the septal surface of the rudimentary chamber. In one further heart, however, although the bundle was posterior, conducting fibers were not found within the rudimentary chamber.

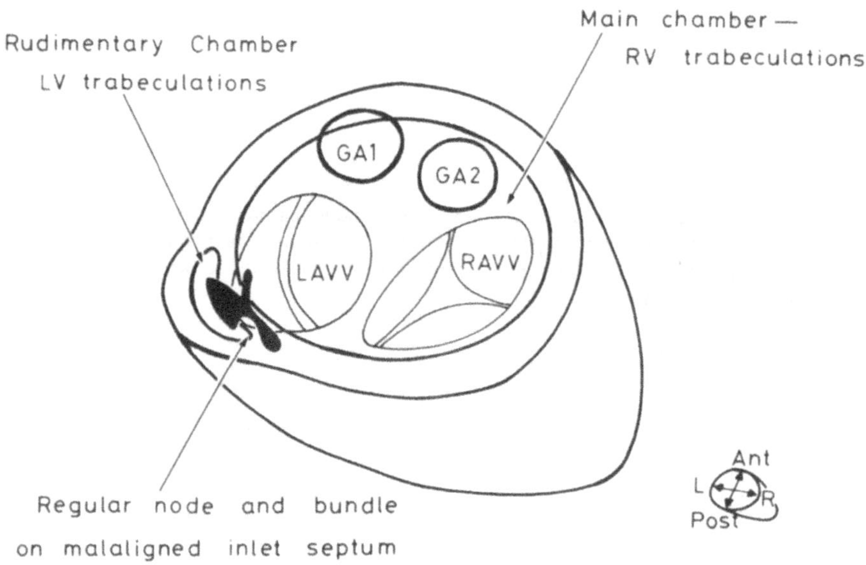

Figure 13. Diagram illustrating the disposition of conducting tissue in univentricular heart of right ventricular type with rudimentary chamber and double inlet.

Two hearts have been examined in which hearts with ventricular morphology of right ventricle and right sided rudimentary chamber were associated with absence of the right atrioventricular connexion and straddling of the left atrioventricular valve. In both hearts, two atrioventricular connexions were identified. The anterior connexion was from the floor of the blind ending right atrium. The posterior connexion was in the posterior wall of the left atrium. The two penetrating bundles joined together to form a sling on the inferior margin of the defect in the inlet septum. A right bundle branch

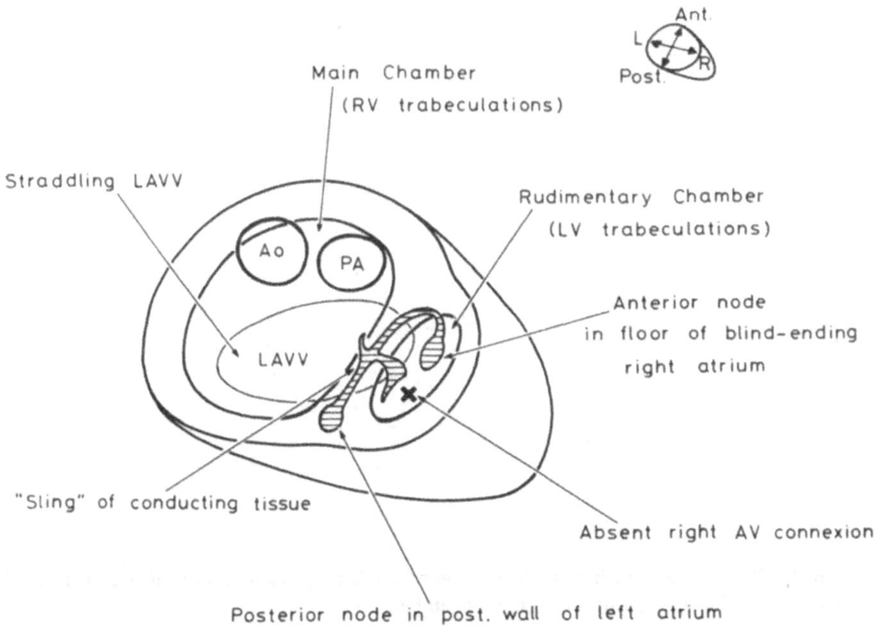

Figure 14. Diagram illustrating the unusual disposition of conducting tissue in three hearts we have studied with univentricular heart of right ventricular type, right sided rudimentary chamber, absent right atrioventricular connexion and straddling left atrioventricular valve. These hearts can be considered as a variant of corrected transposition with 'mitral atresia', but they present as absent right atrioventricular connexion. The conducting tissue has been constant in all three hearts studied.

supplied the main chamber and typical left bundle branch fibers were identified in the rudimentary chamber of left ventricular type (fig. 14).

c) without rudimentary chamber

Four such hearts have been examined, all with double inlet to the sole ventricular chamber (10). In all hearts a posterior node has been found in the base of the atrial septum which did not effect atrioventricular connexion. The connecting atrioventricular bundle originated from an anteriorly situated atrioventricular node. The penetrating bundle in two hearts ran directly into the lateral margin of the ventricular mass, ramifying as it did so (fig. 15). In the other two hearts the bundle passed from an anterior node onto a free-running trabecula. It descended on the trabecula to the ventricular apex, where it ramified into the ventricular myocardium.

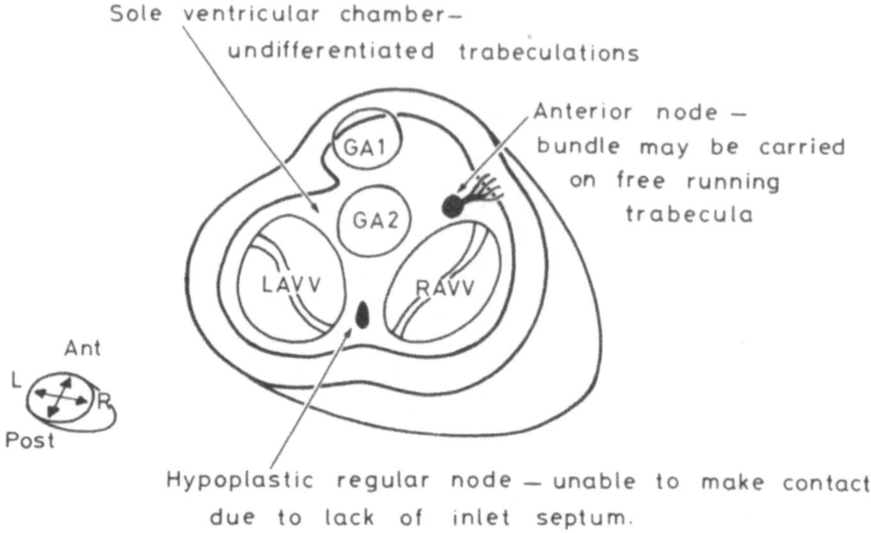

Figure 15. Diagram illustrating the disposition of conducting tissue in univentricular heart of undifferentiated type without rudimentary chamber.

d) Huge Ventricular Septal Defect

Some authorities classify hearts with right ventricular trabeculae to one side and left ventricular myocardium to the other side of a ventricular cavity as examples of univentricular heart (1). In our experience, the only hearts we have seen of this type have also possessed remnants of both the inlet and trabecular septa. Although we initially classified them as primitive ventricles (10), we now believe we were mistaken, and that they are better classified as huge septal defects. As may be anticipated, because the inlet septum is present it carried the conducting tissue in both the hearts we studied, the bundle descending posterior to the defect from a normally situated connecting atrioventricular node (fig. 16).

COMMENT

The key to the disposition of the conducting tissue is the inlet septum. In nearly all the hearts in which this septum is absent, that is in univentricular hearts of left ventricular type or univentricular hearts without a rudimentary chamber, the connecting atrioventricular node is located in antero-lateral

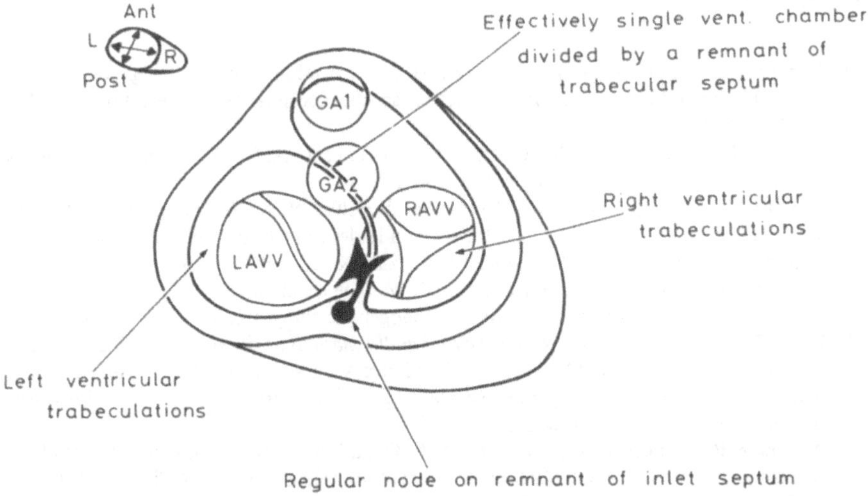

Figure 16. Diagram illustrating the disposition of conducting tissue in hearts with a huge ventricular septal defect. Some authorities classify these hearts as a variant of the univentricular heart ('common ventricle'). We would prefer to classify them as atrioventricular concordance (or discordance) with huge ventricular septal defect.

position. In contrast, when the inlet septum is present, as in univentricular hearts of right ventricular type or huge ventricular septal defects, it carries the connecting atrioventricular bundle. It is important to make these distinctions prior to operating on univentricular hearts, since such knowledge will enable the location of the bundle to be predicted with a high degree of accuracy. However, the bundle location *cannot* be predicted with certainty, and it is our opinion that surgery in the univentricular heart should only be performed when electrophysiological location of the bundle is possible. The heart most likely to be operated on is the univentricular heart of left ventricular type with a rudimentary chamber which supports the aorta. Our studies show that the disposition of the conducting tissue in this anomaly is dependant upon the position of the outlet chamber. In all hearts, the connecting node is at the acute margin of the right atrioventricular orifice. However, in hearts with a left sided outlet chamber, the bundle encircles the pulmonary outflow tract to reach the anterior margin of the trabecular septum. In contrast, with a right sided outlet chamber the bundle descends directly to the posterior margin of the septum, being some distance from the pulmonary valve (fig. 7).

REFERENCES

1. Van Praagh, R., Ongley, P. A. and Swan, H. J. C., Anatomic types of single or common ventricle in man. Morphologic and geometric aspects of 60 necropsied cases. *Am. J. Cardiol.* 13, 367 (1964).
2. Lev, M., Liberthson, R. R., Kirkpatrick, J. R., Eckner, F. A. O. and Arcilla, R. A., Single (primitive) ventricle. *Circulation* 39, 577 (1969).
3. Bharati, S., McAllister, H. A., Jr., Tatooles, C. J., Miller, R. A., Weinberg, M., Bucheleres, H. G. and Lev, M., Anatomic variations in underdeveloped right ventricle related to tricuspid atresia and stenosis. *J. Thorac. Cardiovasc. Surg.* 72, 383 (1976).
4. Goor, D. A., Edwards, J. E. and Lillehei, C. W., The development of the interventricular septum of the human heart; correlative morphogenetic study. *Chest* 58, 453 (1970).
5. Goor, D. A. and Lillehei, C. W., *Congenital malformations of the heart.* New York 1975.
6. Quero-Jimenez, M., Perez Martinez, V. M., Maitre Azcarate, M. J., Merino Batres, G. and Moreno-Granados, R., Exaggerated displacement of the Atrioventricular Canal towards the Bulbus Cordis. *Br. Heart J.* 35, 65 (1973).
7. Anderson, R. H., Becker, A. E., Wenink, A. C. G. and Janse, M. J., The development of the cardiac specialized tissue. In: *The Conduction System of the Heart.* Eds. Wellens, H. J. J., Lie, K. I. and Janse, M. J., Leiden 1976.
8. Wenink, A. C. G., Development of the human cardiac conducting system. *J. Anat.* 121, 617 (1976).
9. Anderson, R. H., Arnold, R., Thapar, M. K., Jones, R. S. and Hamilton, D. I., Cardiac Specialized Tissue in Hearts with an apparently Single Ventricular Chamber (Double Inlet Left Ventricle). *Am. J. Cardiol.* 33, 95 (1974).
10. Wilkinson, J. L., Anderson, R. H., Arnold, R., Hamilton, D. I. and Smith, A., The conducting tissues in primitive ventricular hearts without an outlet chamber. *Circulation* 53, 930 (1976).

ACKNOWLEDGEMENTS

We are greatly indebted to our various colleagues who have contributed markedly to many of the concepts outlined in this chapter, particularly Drs. M. J. Tynan; E. A. Shinebourne and L. M. Gerlis and Prof. F. J. Macartney. We are indebted by Mrs. A. Smith and Mrs. S. Y. Ho for their considerable technical assistance and to Miss Noelle de Freitas for help in the preparation of the manuscript.

8. THE ATRIOVENTRICULAR CONDUCTION TISSUES IN CONGENITALLY CORRECTED TRANSPOSITION

A. E. BECKER AND R. H. ANDERSON

INTRODUCTION

Congenitally corrected transposition is a cardiac malformation characterized by the combined occurrence of a *dis*cordant connection between atria and ventricles and a *dis*cordant connection between the ventricles and the great arteries. In other words, the right atrium connects to the morphological left ventricle from which the pulmonary trunk arises, while the left atrium connects to the morphological right ventricle from which the aorta arises. From a point of view of flow pattern the 'transposition' of the great arteries, in the sense of an aorta arising from the morphological right ventricle, seems corrected by the discordant atrioventricular connection, since systemic and pulmonic venous blood are still conveyed to their proper arterial systems.

This congenital malformation may occur with either a situs solitus or a situs inversus morphology of the atria (fig. 1), which in earlier reports has led to the distinction of a 'bulboventricular' and a 'sinu-atrial' corrected type, respectively (for an extensive review of the literature see Losekoot (1)).

THE ATRIOVENTRICULAR CONDUCTION TISSUES

It has long been recognized that in congenitally corrected transposition the morphology of the ventricular bundle branches followed that of the ventricles (2-5). In the most common condition, with a situs solitus morphology of the atria, the bundle branches showed an inverted morphology in that fan-like left bundle branches were present on the ventricular septal surface on the right, in accord with the 'inverted' position of the morphological left ventricle. However, there is no common consent with respect to the course of the penetrating bundle, connecting the atrioventricular node to the ventricular bundle branches. In 1963, Lev, Licata and May (6) documented a left-sided position of the atrioventricular node in a heart with congenitally corrected transpo-

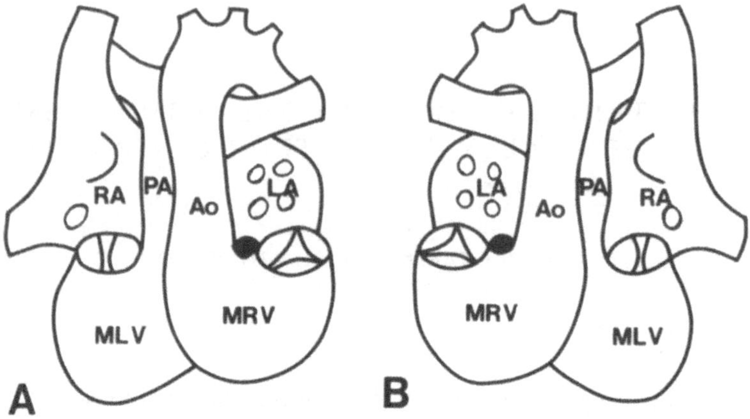

Figure 1. Schematic drawing of the heart with congenitally corrected transposition. The condition may occur with either a situs solitus (A) or a situs inversus (B) morphology of the atria. Basically the heart exhibits a discordant atrioventricular connection, i.e. the right atrium (RA) connects to the morphological left ventricle (MLV) and the left atrium (LA) connects to the morphological right ventricle (MRV), and a discordant ventriculo-arterial connection, i.e. the morphological left ventricle connects to the pulmonary artery (PA) and the morphological right ventricle to the aorta (Ao).

sition and 'solitus atria', while the bundle descended onto the ventricular septum closely related to the left posterior border of the membranous septum. This report is of particular interest since the bundle continued anteriorly, even after all bundle branches had separated, to eventually run out of the block used for histological study. At the same time in 1963, Lev, Fielding and Zaeske (7) described another specimen with congenitally corrected transposition in which they demonstrated, in addition to a normally right-sided 'posterior' node, an abnormally positioned atrioventricular node in the anterior margin of the right atrioventricular orifice. This particular report, however, received much less attention than the one previously quoted.

The important issue of the precise position of the node and penetrating bundle was revived by Anderson and co-workers in 1973 (8) and 1974 (9) in documenting an anterior node from which the penetrating bundle originated. These findings actually endorsed the documentation of an anterior node and bundle by Uher (10) in 1936; a report which since then has been practically forgotten. The bundle, from its anterior location, descended onto the ventricular myocardium in close relation to the pulmonary outflow tract; a disposition which has important surgical connotations and merits further detailed description.

ANATOMICAL FEATURES OF CONGENITALLY CORRECTED TRANSPOSITION RELEVANT TO THE ATRIOVENTRICULAR CONDUCTION TISSUES

For the basic understanding of the disposition of the atrioventricular conduction tissues in congenitally corrected transposition there are two main features that need to be evaluated.

Firstly, it is important to realize that in these hearts the atrial septum and the inlet portion of the interventricular septum may no longer be well appositioned. Indeed, when closely observed it becomes apparent that in most hearts with a situs solitus morphology of the atria the two septa disperse along their anticipated line of junction (fig. 2A). Posteriorly, at the crux of the heart, the two septa are well aligned but in an anterior direction the two septa separate with the atrial septum deviating rightward relative to the plane of the ventricular inlet septum. This anatomical feature may have a major impact upon the possibilities for a normally positioned atrioventricular node to actually contact ventricular myocardium. A descending bundle from such a node may find no ventricular septum underneath to descend upon. Indeed, most hearts with a solitus morphology of atria, thusfar studied histologically, although exhibiting an atrioventricular node in its usual position, had no contacting bundle in that location. However, it is fundamental in this concept to realize that possibility or impossibility for a node to descend will depend upon the degree of 'malalignment' between the two septa. Since this degree may vary from one case to another, one should be prepared to accept the possibility of a 'normal' descending bundle, although such an occasion in our experience is an exception rather than the rule.

The second anatomical feature of paramount importance is the deeply wedged position of the pulmonic ostium, between the two atrioventricular ostia (fig. 2). Because of the deviating cardiac septa, the pulmonic ostium viewed from the morphologic left ventricle is more or less hidden underneath the large septal leaflet of the 'inverted' mitral valve (fig. 2B). The precise localization of the pulmonic ostium relative to the atrial septum, the right atrial orifice and the ventricular septum is significant with regard to the alternative route that a descending atrioventricular bundle may take. In order to fully appreciate such a disposition of the conduction tissues one should be familiar with the fact that the atrioventricular node and bundle develop in situ from anlagen which embryologically present as rings of 'specialized' tissues encircling the atrioventricular and ventriculo-bulbar junction (11, 12). The right atrioventricular ring tissue, from which a major part of the compact

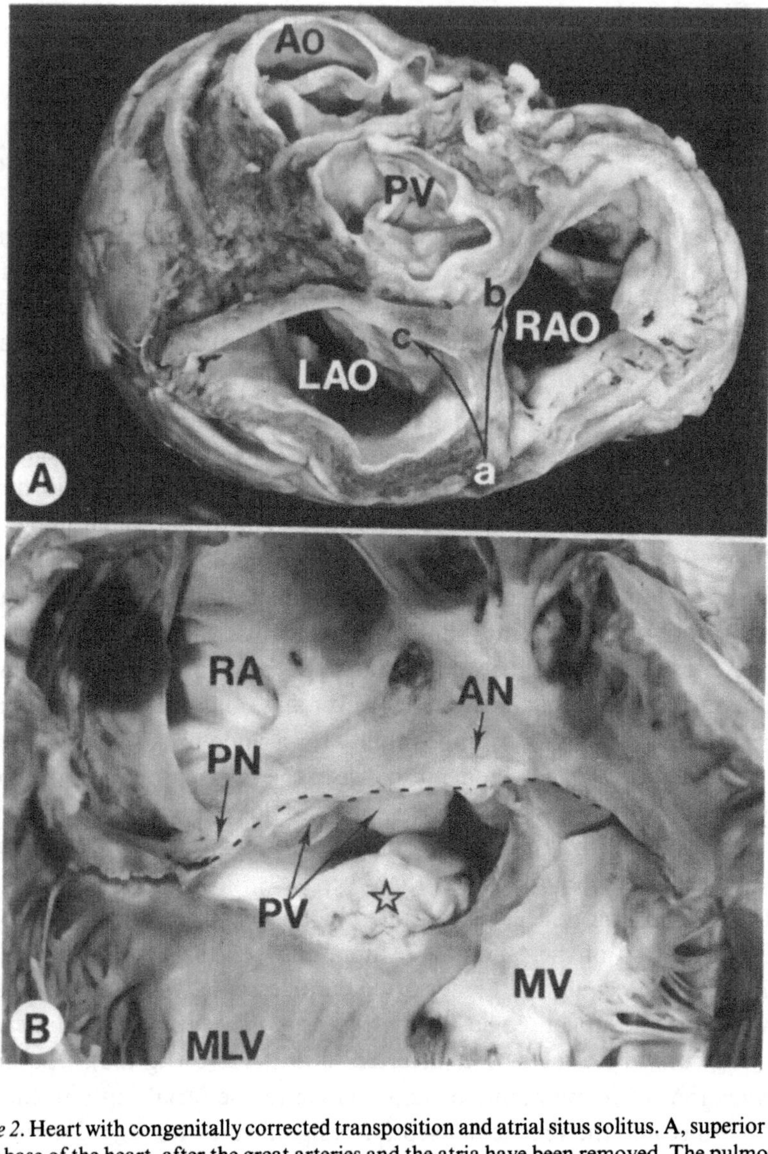

Figure 2. Heart with congenitally corrected transposition and atrial situs solitus. A, superior view of the base of the heart, after the great arteries and the atria have been removed. The pulmonary valve (PV) is posterior relative to the aorta (Ao), wedged between the right (RAO) and left atrial orifices (LAO). This superior view demonstrates the malalignment between the atrial septum (a-b) and the inlet portion of the ventricular septum (a-c). Both septa join at the crux of the heart (a) but in an anterior direction the two septa disperse with the atrial septum positioned to the right, relative to the underlying ventricular septum. B, detailed view of the junction between the right atrium (RA) and the morphological left ventricle (MLV) viewed from the right side. In order to visualize the deeply positioned pulmonic valve (PV) the 'inverted' septal leaflet of the mitral valve

atrioventricular node develops, normally shows a node-like expansion in its anterior segment. Remnants of this expansion may persist throughout development into the mature heart, albeit that such remnants normally will not contact ventricular myocardium (13). It is our belief that the description by Kent (14) of a node-like structure in the lateral right atrial wall actually represented this remnant. However, we disagree with his interpretation that this structure normally connects atrial to ventricular myocardium. Nevertheless, in congenital cardiac malformations with absent or abnormal cardiac septational processes, the ring tissues and in particular the 'anterior node' may persist and may give rise to an atrioventricular node and penetrating bundle. This concept can explain the disposition of the conduction tissues in the univentricular hearts of left ventricular and indeterminate types, and it may also explain the disposition encountered in congenitally corrected transposition. Because of the malalignment of the atrial septum with respect to the inlet portion of the ventricular septum, the posterior node may be unable to contact ventricular myocardium and the anterior part of the atrioventricular ring tissue may develop into an accessory node from which the penetrating bundle may descend onto the ventricular myocardium. However, the descending bundle will then be in close contact with the pulmonic outflow tract and actually will encircle its anterior segment before descending onto the ventricular septum. In other words, we contend that the disposition of the atrioventricular conduction tissues in congenitally corrected transposition relates to the peculiar anatomical situation of (1) malaligned cardiac septa and (2) the wedged position of the pulmonic ostium relative to the right atrial orifice.

SURGICAL ANATOMY OF THE ATRIOVENTRICULAR NODE AND PENETRATING BUNDLE

Most experience has thusfar been gained in hearts with a situs solitus morphology of the atria; the most common form of congenitally corrected trans-

(MV) has been cut loose from its basal attachment (dotted line). A fibrous tissue tag (asterisk) is present underneath the pulmonic valve accounting for subvalvar pulmonic stenosis. The positions of the posterior (PN) and anterior atrioventricular nodes (AN) are indicated. The area directly underneath the posterior node is formed by that part of the membranous septum, which intervenes between left atrium and the morphological left ventricle. A bundle, therefore, cannot descend upon the ventricular septum. The anterior node, on the other hand, may descend upon the anterior part of the interventricular septum (compare to figures 3A and B).

position. In these hearts two atrioventricular nodes can be anticipated. The first one will be positioned in its usual position, delineated by the tendon of Todaro (fig. 2B). In our experience, however, this node will only rarely possess a penetrating bundle contacting ventricular myocardium (9). Of 11 hearts studied histologically only one case had a posterior bundle, originating from a 'posterior' node. However, all 11 hearts in this series possessed an anterior

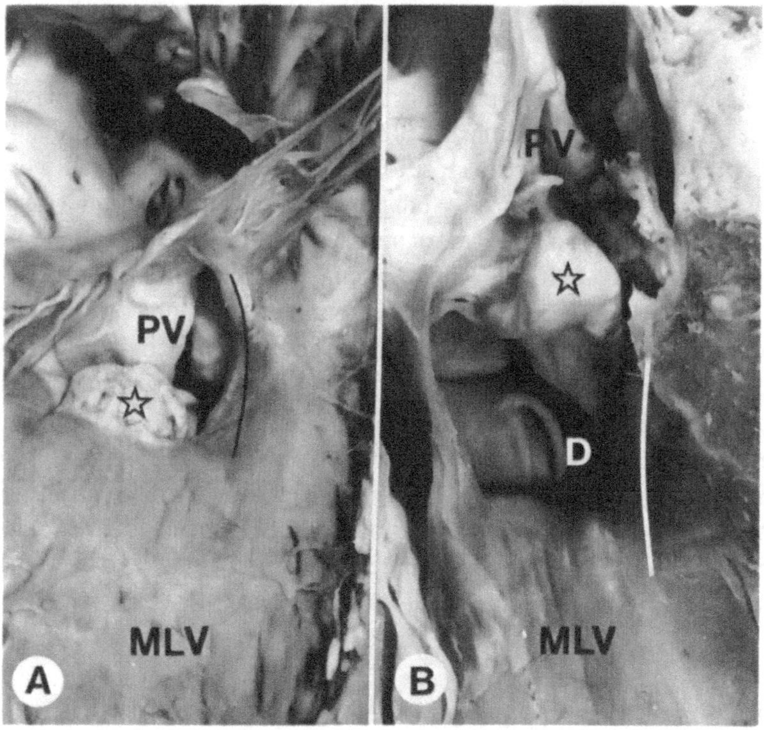

Figure 3. Two specimens of congenitally corrected transposition with atrial situs solitus, in which the outflow tract of the morphological left ventricle (MLV) has been exposed. The course of the penetrating bundle, originating from the anterior node (compare to figure 2B), is schematically indicated by a solid line. A, (same specimen as illustrated in figure 2B). This specimen exihibited *no* ventricular septal defect. The anterior contacting bundle descends close to the pulmonic valve (PV), along the right anterior margin of the pulmonary outflow tract. There is no direct relationship between the bundle and the fibrous tissue tag (asterisk) obstructing the outflow tract. B, Specimen with a subvalvar ventricular septal defect (D) and pulmonary stenosis due to an aneurysmal tissue tag (asterisk), derived from the interventricular part of the membranous septum, located directly underneath the pulmonary valve (PV). The bundle descends onto the ventricular septum along the anterior border of the defect; a location opposite to that anticipated in isolated ventricular septal defect.

node from which the penetrating bundle originated. In other words, in one instance a posterior *and* anterior penetrating bundle was present. The anterior node is located in the base of the atrial wall, just anterior and lateral to the interatrial septum and central fibrous body (fig. 2B). The bundle in this position will penetrate the anulus fibrosus and will reach the ventricle subendocardially in the anterior wall of the pulmonic outflow tract close to the pulmonary valve (fig. 3). The bundle will course along the anterior margin of the pulmonary outflow tract to reach the interventricular septum and will then descend towards the apex giving rise to both left and right bundle branches (fig. 3A). In case of a subvalvar ventricular septal defect, the bundle

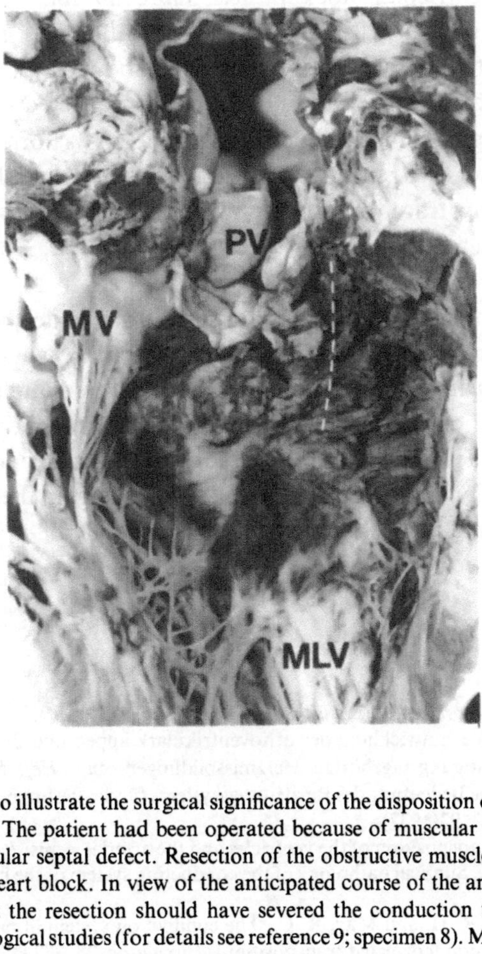

Figure 4. Specimen to illustrate the surgical significance of the disposition of the atrioventricular conduction bundle. The patient had been operated because of muscular subpulmonic stenosis and a small ventricular septal defect. Resection of the obstructive muscle mass had led to immediate complete heart block. In view of the anticipated course of the anterior bundle (dotted line) it is clear that the resection should have severed the conduction tissues; a supposition confirmed by histological studies (for details see reference 9; specimen 8). MLV = morphological left ventricle; MV = mitral valve; PV = pulmonic valve.

will descend along the anterior border of the defect (fig. 3B); a position, therefore, quite opposite to the anticipated localization in isolated ventricular septal defect.

The course of the atrioventricular bundle is of particular surgical significance, since congenitally corrected transposition is frequently complicated by pulmonic outflow tract stenoses, either valvar or subvalvar, and subvalvar ventricular septal defects (15, 16). In each of these circumstances surgical repair may easily jeopardize the atrioventricular conduction bundle because of its intimate relationship with each of these structures (fig. 4). Moreover, the bundle takes an attenuated course rendering it vulnerable to processes of wear and tear, which may explain the high frequency of naturally occurring atrioventricular block in these malformations.

In hearts with congenitally corrected transposition and situs inversus morphology of the atria, we are less well informed about the precise course of the penetrating bundle. However, the data thusfar collected seem to indicate a preference for a posterior atrioventricular node, in its normal position albeit 'inverted', from which a posterior connecting bundle arises. In some instances the bundle has been traced anteriorly, but direct contact with an anterior node has as yet not been established.

In *summary*, the data thusfar collected seem to indicate that in hearts with congenitally corrected transposition and a situs solitus morphology of the atria, an anterior node with an anterior penetrating bundle seems the rule, although a posterior connecting node may occasionally be present also.

In cases with a situs inversus morphology of the atria a posterior connecting atrioventricular node seems to be the rule, but again the possibility of an anterior connecting node should always be considered.

REFERENCES

1. Losekoot, G., *Gecorrigeerde Transposities*. Thesis Amsterdam 1967.
2. Sato, S., Über die Entwicklung der atrioventrikularklappen und der pars membranacea unter Berücksichtigung zugehöriger Herzmissbildungen. *Anat. Heft.* 50, 195 (1914).
3. Aschoff, J. L., Die Bedeutung des Reizleitungssystems für die Bestimmung der Herzfehler. *J. Tech. Methods* 17, 93(1937).
4. Walmsley, T., Transposition of the ventricles and the arterial stems. *J. Anat.* 65, 528 (1930).
5. Hudson, R. E. B., Surgical pathology of the conducting system of the heart. *Br. Heart J.* 29, 646 (1967).
6. Lev, M., Licata, R. H. and May, R. C., The conduction system in mixed levocardia with ventricular inversion (corrected transposition). *Circulation* 28, 232 (1963).

7. Lev, M., Fielding, R. T. and Zaeske, D., Mixed levocardia with ventricular inversion (corrected transposition) with complete atrioventricular block. *Am. J. Cardiol.* 12, 875 (1963).
8. Anderson, R. H., Arnold, R. and Wilkinson, J. L., The conducting system in classically corrected transposition. *Lancet* 1, 1286 (1973).
9. Anderson, R. H., Becker, A. E., Arnold, R. and Wilkinson, J. L., The conducting tissues in congenitally corrected transposition. *Circulation* 50, 911 (1974).
10. Uher, V., Zur Pathologie des Reizleitungssystems bei kongenitalen Herzanomalien. *Frankf. Z. Pathol.* 49, 347 (1936).
11. Anderson, R. H., Becker, A. E., Wenink, A. C. G. and Janse, M. J., The development of the cardiac specialized tissue. In: Wellens, H. J. J., et al. (ed.), *The Conduction System of the Heart.* Leiden 1976.
12. Wenink, A. C. G., Development of the human cardiac conducting system. *J. Anat.* 121, 617 (1976).
13. Anderson, R. H., Davies, M. J. and Becker, A. E., Atrioventricular ring specialized tissue in the normal heart. *Eur. J. Cardiol.* 2, 219 (1974).
14. Kent, A. F. S., The right lateral auriculo-ventricular junction of the heart. *J. Physiol.* 48, 22 (1914).
15. Anderson, R. H., Becker, A. E. and Gerlis, L. M., The pulmonary outflow tract in classically corrected transposition. *J. Thorac. Cardiovasc. Surg.* 69, 747 (1975).
16. Allwork, S. P., Bentall, H. H., Becker, A. E., Cameron, H., Gerlis, L. M., Wilkinson, J. L. and Anderson, R. H., Congenitally corrected transposition of the great arteries: morphologic study of 32 cases. *Am. J. Cardiol.* 38, 910 (1976).

PART II

TRANSPOSITION OF THE GREAT ARTERIES

A. Pathogenesis

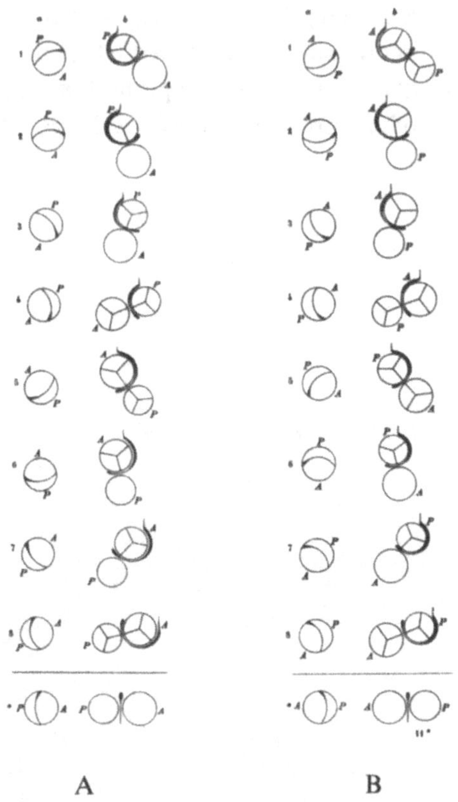

Figure 2. Reproduction of Figures 40 and 42 from 'Die Defekte der Scheidewände des Herzens' by Rokitansky (9). He explained the various positions of the great arteries which produced 'corrected' (scheme A) or 'transposed' (scheme B) circulations on the direction of growth and convexity of the truncal septum (the 'tadpole' in each figure).

arterial discordance. They argued that if the conotruncal septum was formed in straight rather than spiral fashion, then the systemic component of the aortic arch system would become connected to the right rather than the left ventricle. Van Mierop and his colleagues (11-13) again focused attention on the truncus, but proposed a different mechanism for production of ventriculo-arterial discordance. They had clearly described the series of anomalies consisting of ventricular septal defect, Eisenmenger's complex, tetralogy of Fallot and double outlet right ventricle with sub-aortic defect.

They pointed out that a common denominator of this series was faulty transfer of the posterior great artery. However, they considered that production of ventriculo-arterial discordance was unrelated either to infundibular maldevelopment or to formation of a straight septum. Instead, they opined that it resulted from fusion of inappropriate truncal swellings with the conal septum (fig. 3).

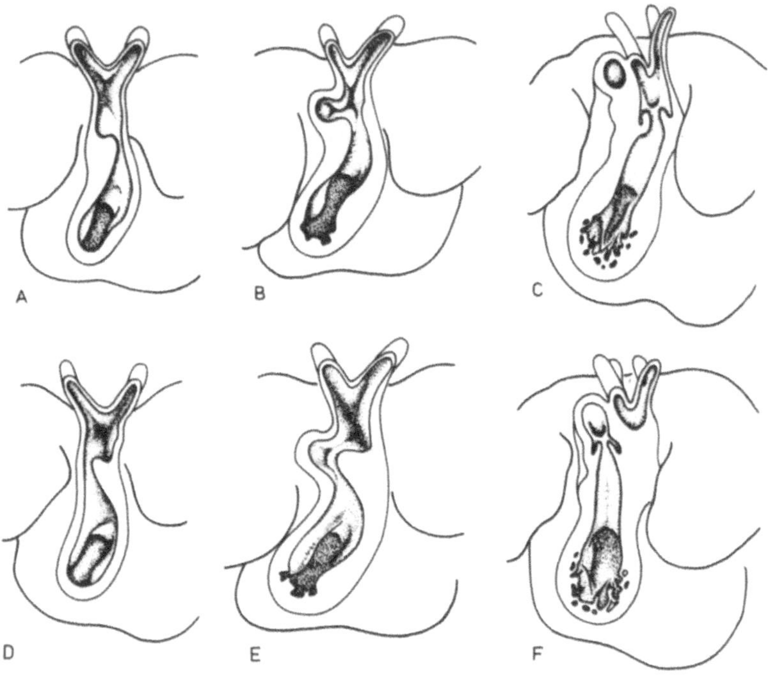

Figure 3. Drawing of Figure 2 from Van Mierop and Wiglesworth, 1963 (Reference 13). It illustrates normal development of the truncal swellings in diagrams A through C, showing how the pulmonary arteries are connected to the right ventricular outflow tract. The authors proposed that with reversal of the roles played by truncal and intercalated valve swellings (diagrams D through F) the *aorta* could become connected to the right ventricular outflow tract. Reproduced by permission of Dr. L. H. S. Van Mierop and the American Journal of Cardiology.

More recently interest has again returned to the infundibular region as the 'factory' for ventriculo-arterial discordance. This is largely due to the writings of Van Praagh and his associates (14-19). The evidence for their concept is well summarized by Paul, Van Praagh and Van Praagh (16). These authors pointed out that *anatomical* evidence contended against truncal malseptation

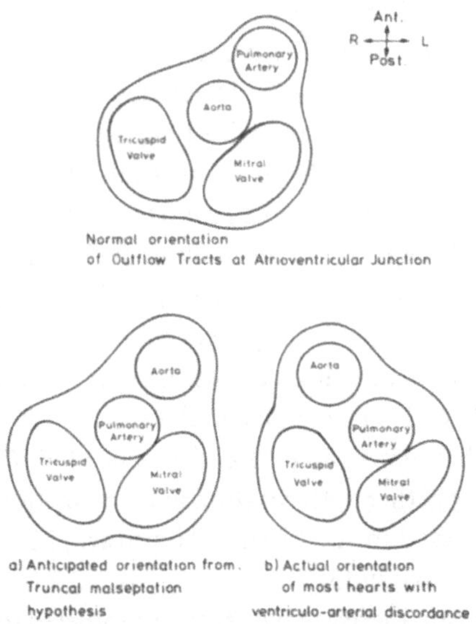

Figure 4. Diagrams illustrating the concept underlying the conal maldevelopment of hypothesis of Van Praagh and his colleagues (15, 16). The upper diagram illustrates the normal orientation of the arterial valves as viewed from below. Van Praagh et al. argued that truncal malseptation should produce arterial orientation as shown in figure 4a. However, their anatomical studies showed that this was not the case, the arteries in 'transposition' being orientated as in figure 4b.

theories as the cause of ventriculo-arterial discordance. They argued that if the truncal septum 'plugged' the aorta into the wrong outflow tract, as suggested by the truncal malseptationists, then the aortic infundibulum in ventriculo-arterial discordance should resemble the pulmonary infundibulum in the normal heart (fig. 4a). However, in the material they had studied, the aortic infundibulum in ventriculo-arterial discordance was invariably a right sided structure (fig. 4b). Because of this anatomic evidence, they proposed their conal growth hypothesis to account for ventriculo-arterial discordance. They had considered a conal absorption hypothesis, but felt that embryological evidence then extant did not support this concept, although they indicated that Butler (20) had demonstrated the importance of conal absorption in the chick heart. In fact, Pernkopf and Wirtinger (21) had also noted the importance of absorption of the bulbar region of the heart during the normal transfer of the aorta to the definitive left ventricle. This work was subsequently confirmed by Asami (22). Its significance to the genesis of ventriculo-arterial discordance was stressed by Goor and his colleagues (23, 24). They pointed out the vital role of conal rotation in addition to conal absorption and showed how these two factors could account for the genesis of the spectrum of anomalies previously described by Lev and Saphir (6). In the meantime, this spectrum had been described again by Lev and his colleagues (25), Lev himself, writing with Eckner (26) had earlier suggested that the spectrum could result from incorporation of the sub-pulmonary bulbar area into the left ventricle. The importance of bulbar absorption together with abnormal rotation of the bulbus during development was endorsed by our own studies (27, 28). We suggested also the possible importance of rightward deviation of the anterior part of the interventricular septum. The spectrum of anomalies from double outlet right ventricle to ventriculo-arterial discordance had also been noted and their embryogenetic significance discussed by Quero-Jimenez et al. (29) and Thiene et al. (30). Over the same period this spectrum together with rotation and absorption of the bulbus had been extensively discussed in the German literature, notably by Doerr (31-33), Bersch (34) and Chuaqui (35).

In summary, therefore, there are two basic hypotheses regarding genesis of ventriculo-arterial discordance. On the one hand some authorities argue that the anomaly results from disordered growth of the infundibular region of the heart and that a spectrum exists between the anomalies of double outlet right ventricle and ventriculo-arterial discordance. In contrast, others argue that double outlet and ventriculo-arterial discordance are unrelated in morphogenetic terms, and that ventriculo-arterial discordance results from abnormal septation of the truncal region of the heart.

EVIDENCE FROM NORMAL DEVELOPMENT PERTINENT TO THE GENESIS OF VENTRICULO-ARTERIAL DISCORDANCE

It is known that following formation of the primary heart tube, the bulbo-truncal junction is separated from the atrioventricular junction by the entirety of the ventricular and bulbar segments of the tube. Following ventriculo-bulbar looping, these segments achieve inner and outer curvatures. It is then the inner curvature of the tube which effectively separates the atrioventricular and bulbo-truncal junctions (fig. 5). Since the arterial valves are formed at the bulbo-truncal junction, and the atrioventricular valves at the atrioventricular junction, it is evident that at this early stage the presumptive valve sites are separated by the inner curvature, which may be termed the ventriculo-infundibular fold. Since the division of the bulbus by the bulbar endocardial cushions, produces the presumptive outflow tracts it is also evident that both

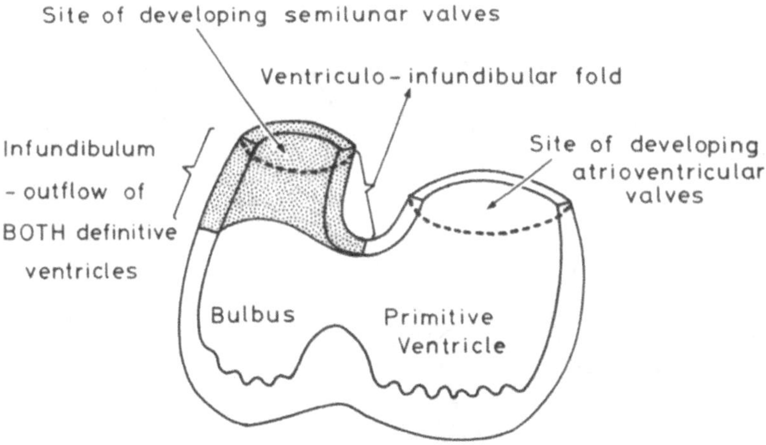

Figure 5. Diagram showing the morphology of the ventriculobulbar segments of the heart tube after looping. Note that the developing arterial and atrioventricular valves are separated by the inner curvature, and that initially a segment of infundibulum is present beneath both developing arterial valves.

tracts are supported by the bulbus. There is considerable evidence from the studies of Van Mierop et al. (11) and Goor, Dische and Lillehei (25) that rotation of the bulbus occurs during the looping process, so that the right sided part of the distal bulbus becomes posterior relative to the left sided part (fig. 6). This process can be termed normal rotation of the distal bulbus. The studies of Pernkopf and Wirtinger (23), Goerttler (38), Van Mierop et al. (11), Asami (24), Goor et al. (25) and Anderson et al. (29) have all shown that normal development of the ventricular outflow tracts then occurs by transfer of the posterior, right sided aortic infundibulum to the left ventricle. During this transfer there is attenuation of the mid-portion of the ventriculo-infundibular fold so that the developing aortic valve is brought into continuity with the mitral valve. In terms of absolute growth, the aortic outflow tract obviously increases in size with subsequent development. However, in terms of development events, the evidence is overwhelming that the developing aortic outflow tract originates above the bulbus as a complete myoblastic infundibulum and becomes relatively decreased in size as it is transferred to the left ventricle.

With regard to truncal development, Van Mierop and his colleagues (11) identified separate conal and truncal swellings as being of significance in cono-truncal septation. The studies of Los (39) suggested that these swellings

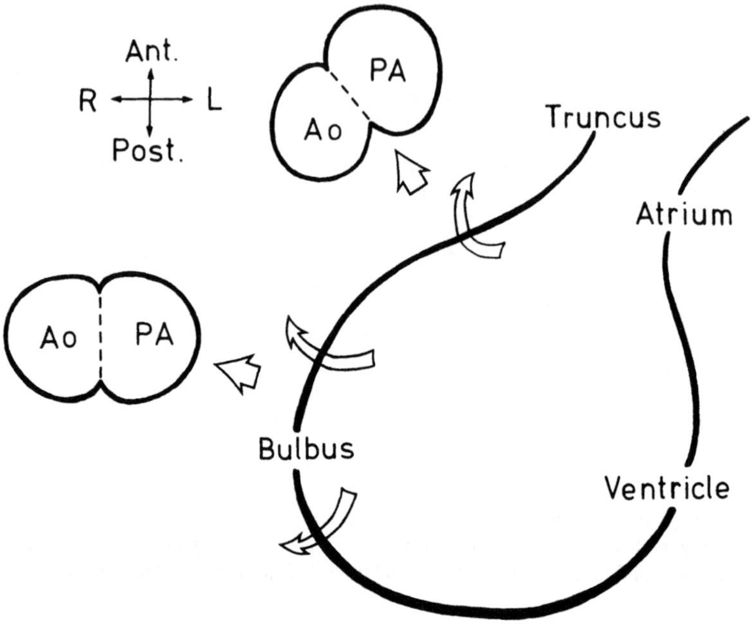

Figure 6. Diagram illustrating how the looping process itself imparts torsion to the bulbar component. When viewed from beneath (see 'weather-vane' for orientation) this torsion brings the presumptive aortic outflow tract to a right posterior position (Ao - aorta; PA - pulmonary artery).

were continuous bulbo-truncal structures, but he demonstrated the importance of the aortico-pulmonary septum in truncal septation. This structure originated from the junction of the fourth and sixth arches in the aortic sac, but then grew proximally towards the truncus, fusing with the bulbo-truncal swellings to complete the septation process. Los's reconstructions additionally showed another vital facet of truncal development. Although when they first appeared, the bulbo-truncal swellings were disposed in spiral fashion, on fusion they produced a *straight* bulbo-truncal septum, spiralling of the great arteries occurring in the area derived from the aortic sac.

Normal development can therefore be summarized in terms of rotation of the distal bulbus during looping, attenuation of the sub-aortic component of the distal bulbus, fusion of the bulbo-truncal ridges to form a straight bulbo-truncal septum and completion of truncal septation by downgrowth of the aortico-pulmonary septum.

EVIDENCE FROM MALFORMED HEARTS RELATIVE TO THE GENESIS OF VENTRICULO-ARTERIAL DISCORDANCE

It is our opinion (28) that study of specimens shows that a spectrum of malformations exists between the normal heart with ventriculo-arterial concordance; the normal heart with ventriculo-arterial concordance, a ventricular septal defect and an overriding aorta; the tetralogy of Fallot and double outlet right ventricle with sub-aortic ventricular septal defect (fig. 7). This process was aptly described by Van Mierop et al. (12) as 'Transfer of the Posterior Great Artery', although they did not subscribe to the concept of a spectrum existing

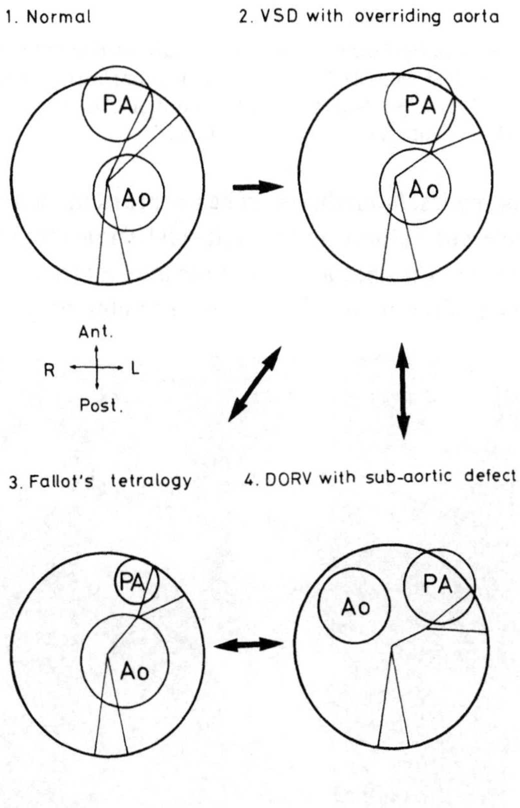

Figure 7. Diagram illustrating the spectrum of malformations which are explained on the basis of failure of transfer of the posterior great artery, in normal development the aorta (Ao). The spectrum stretches from normality (fig. 7.1) through ventricular septal defect (VSD) with overriding aorta (fig. 7.2) to Fallot's tetralogy (also associated with malseptation at the expense of the pulmonary artery (PA), fig. 7.3) and finally to double outlet right ventricle (DORV) with subaortic defect (fig. 7.4).

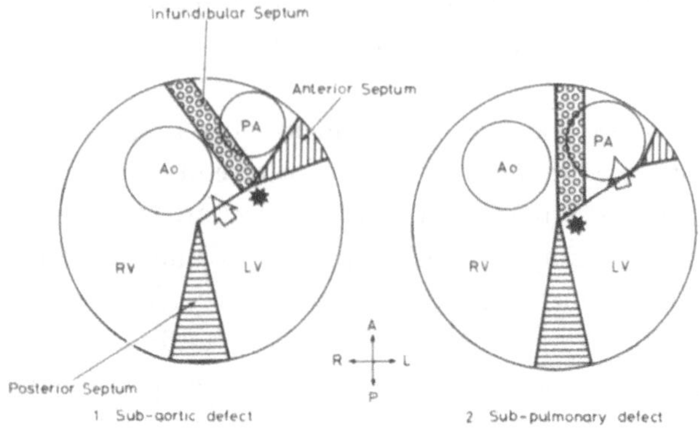

Figure 8. Diagram illustrating how transfer of the septal insertion of the infundibular septum converts double outlet right ventricle (DORV) with sub-aortic (Ao) defect to the same connexion with sub-pulmonary (PA) defect. Note the change in position of the star from the anterior to the posterior septum (RV - right ventricle; LV - left ventricle).

between the anomalies. Nonetheless, if hearts are examined with double outlet right ventricle with sub-aortic defect, it will be noted that the infundibular septum is inserted to the anterior part of the interventricular septum (fig. 8). As a consequence of this mode of insertion, the pulmonary valve is separated

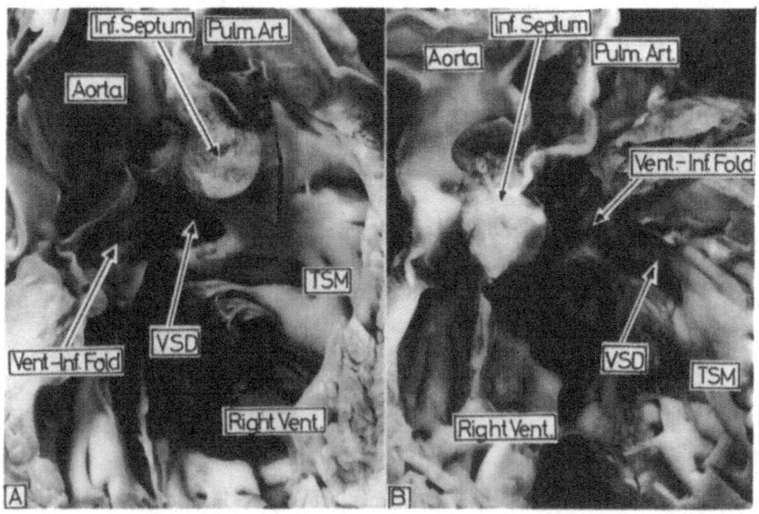

Figure 9. Photographs illustrating transfer of the infundibular (Inf.) septum. Figure 9a shows double outlet right ventricle with sub-aortic defect; Figure 9b shows double outlet right ventricle with sub-pulmonary (Pulm. Art.) defect. Note that the ventriculo-infundibular fold (Vent.-Inf. Fold) and the trabecula septomarginalis (TSM) retain the same relation to the defect (VSD).

from the defect by the infundibular septum. Examination of specimens shows that a further spectrum exists in which the septal insertion of the infundibular septum loses its attachment to the anterior interventricular septum and moves across the ventriculo-infundibular fold before attaching itself to the posterior interventricular septum (fig. 8). This process can be termed 'transfer of the infundibular septum' (28) (fig. 8). It has the effect of transferring the ventricular septal defect in double outlet right ventricle from sub-aortic to sub-pulmonary position (Compare Figures 9a and b). The infundibular septum then separates the aortic valve from the defect, while the pulmonary valve is directly adjacent to the defect. There is then considerable evidence, described initially by Lev and Saphir (6) and subsequently by Lev et al. (25), Goor and Edwards (24) and Anderson et al. (28) that a third spectrum of anomalies exists during which the pulmonary outflow tract is transferred from the right ventricle to the left ventricle, producing ventriculo-arterial discordance. This final transitional series can be termed 'Transfer of the Anterior Great Artery'. It must be emphasized that several morphogenetic events are probably involved in final transfer of the anterior artery to the left ventricle. It can be argued from first principles that there are at least two ways of effecting transfer. The first is to transfer the artery across the septum. The second is to transfer the septum beneath the artery (fig. 10). Evidence from specimens suggests that both these mechanisms probably operate. In the majority of

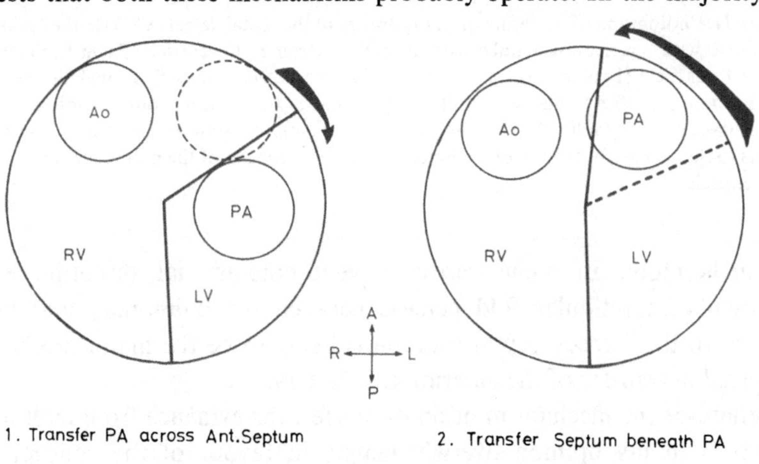

Figure 10. Diagram illustrating how transfer of the anterior artery (the pulmonary artery, PA) can be effected either by movement of the artery across the septum (Figure 10.1) or by transfer of the septum beneath the artery (Figure 10.2). (Ao - aorta; RV - right ventricle; LV - left ventricle; orientation as shown by 'weather-vane').

cases, there is pulmonary-mitral fibrous valvar continuity in ventriculo-arterial discordance, pointing to the role of attenuation of the sub-pulmonary infundibulum (fig. 11). However, the septal role is supported by the fact that the anterior septum in ventriculo-arterial discordance is in line with the posterior septum, unlike the situation in double outlet right ventricle, where the two septal portions subtend a considerable angle to one another (28).

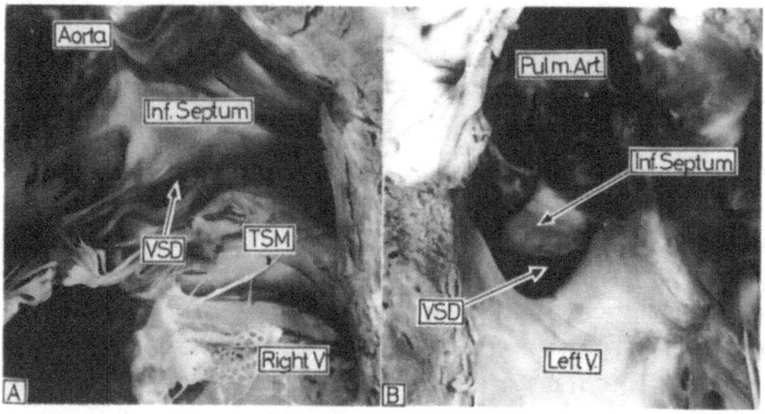

Figure 11. Photographs illustrating the morphology of the septal defect (VSD) in the majority of specimens with ventriculo-arterial discordance. Views from right ventricle (Right V, Figure 11a) and left ventricle (Left V, Figure 11b) show that the defect results from malalignment and malfusion of the infundibular septum (Inf. septum) with the anterior septum, reinforced by the trabecula septomarginalis (TSM). The presence of pulmonary-mitral continuity (Figure 11b) points to the role of absorption of the inner curvature in transfer of the pulmonary artery to the left ventricle.

Furthermore, in some cases of ventriculo-arterial discordance the ventriculo-infundibular fold persists between the pulmonary and mitral valves. In these cases, septal rotation is likely to be the major mechanism involved in transfer of the anterior great artery.

Whatever the mechanism of final transfer, the evidence from malformed hearts is in my opinion overwhelmingly in favour of the concept that ventriculo-arterial discordance with ventricular septal defect is produced by maldevelopment of the infundibular region of the heart.

ARE ALL EXAMPLES OF VENTRICULO-ARTERIAL DISCORDANCE PRODUCED BY INFUNDIBULAR MALDEVELOPMENT?

Although the evidence is in my opinion very strong that hearts with ventricular septal defect and ventriculo-arterial discordance result from infundibular maldevelopment, this does not mean that all hearts with ventriculo-arterial discordance have the same mode of development. Consider the variation in morphology of hearts with ventriculo-arterial discordance. It has already been stated that specimens exist with presence or absence of the subpulmonary ventriculo-infundibular fold. This variation has been explained on the basis of infundibular and ventricular septal maldevelopment. However, there is also considerable variation in arterial interrelationships in ventriculo-arterial discordance. Paul et al. (16) suggested that hearts with ventriculo-arterial discordance invariably had right sided aortic valves. As indicated above, they used this fact as evidence against the truncal malseptation hypothesis. This in itself may not be a valid contention. Van Mierop and Gessner (38) subsequently pointed out that in hearts with ventriculo-arterial concordance and aortic atresia, the pulmonary artery position was directly comparable to the aortic position seen in ventriculo-arterial discordance. They therefore argued that arterial position may be a consequence of secondary haemodynamic influences rather than primary structural maldevelopment. Be that as it may, the assertion is also questionable that aortic position in ventriculo-arterial discordance with situs solitus and atrioventricular concordance is invariably right sided. Carr et al. (39) demonstrated angiographically that in over one hundred successively studied cases, the aortic valve was right sided in less than 70%. In 19% of hearts the aortic outflow tract and valve were left sided, a position directly comparable to the pulmonary position in the normal heart. These findings were subsequently confirmed in a surgical and angiographic study by Lincoln et al. (40). Such hearts with ventriculo-arterial discordance and left sided aortae can exist with or without ventricular septal defects (40). They would be ideally explained on the concept of truncal malseptation, that is growth of the truncal septum so as to 'plug' the developing fourth and sixth arches of the aortic sac into inappropriate outflow tracts (fig. 12). If the morphological evidence suggests that truncal malseptation is a possibility, how then can it be affected? The studies of Los (37, 41) would appear to invalidate the 'straight septum hypothesis' of de la Cruz and Rocha (10), since the normal bulbotruncal septum fuses in straight fashion. Nonetheless, there are still at least two ways in which truncal malseptation could occur. Firstly, as suggested by Van Mierop et al.

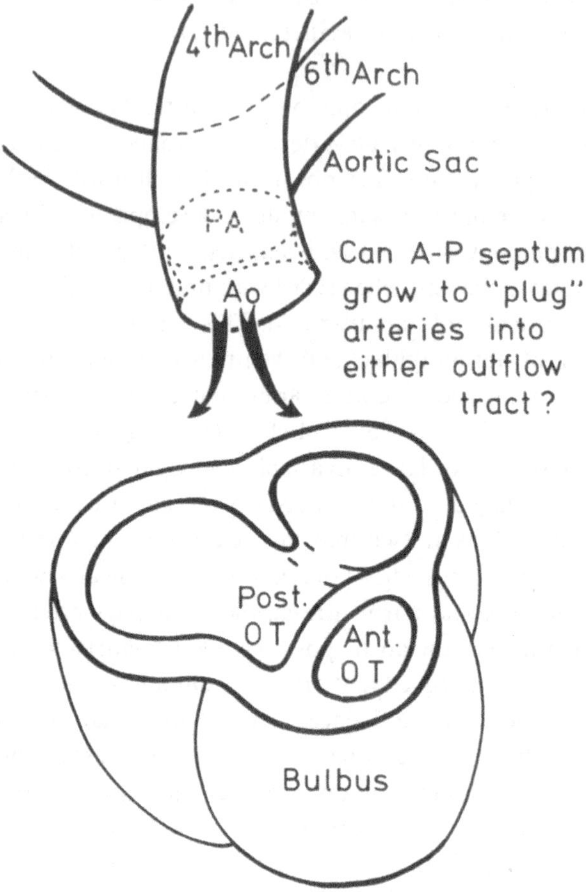

Figure 12. Diagram illustrating the concept of faulty 'plugging-in'. It is possible that the aortico-pulmonary (A - P) septum could grow so as to 'plug' the 4th and 6th arches into either of the developing outflow tracts (post OT; ant. OT).

(11), the 'wrong' truncus swellings could fuse with the bulbar swellings, thus connecting the anterior bulbar outflow tract to the fourth (systemic) arch rather than to the sixth (pulmonary) arch. Alternatively, as suggested by Los (41), the aortico-pulmonary septum may grow down from the aortic sac in reverse so as to produce the same inappropriate 'plugging-in'.

CAN INFUNDIBULAR MALDEVELOPMENT AND TRUNCAL MALSEPTATION CO-EXIST?

Anatomic evidence is consistent with either of the two concepts discussed above being able to produce ventriculo-arterial discordance. However, anatomic evidence also exists to support the hypothesis that both mechanisms can co-exist. It has been described how specimens exist which make up the spectrum of ventriculo-arterial concordance with right posterior aorta; double outlet right ventricle with sub-aortic defect and right sided aorta; double outlet right ventricle with sub-pulmonary defect and right sided aorta and ventriculo-arterial discordance with right sided aorta (fig. 13). It is also

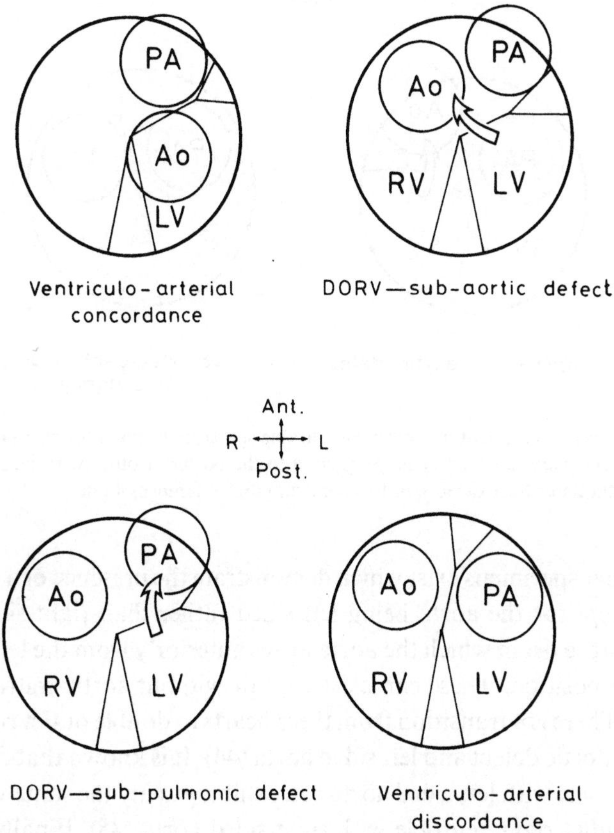

Figure 13. Diagram illustrating the spectrum of malformations known to exist when the aorta is 'plugged' into the posterior outflow tract normally transferred to the left ventricle (LV) - Compare with Figures 7, 8, 10.

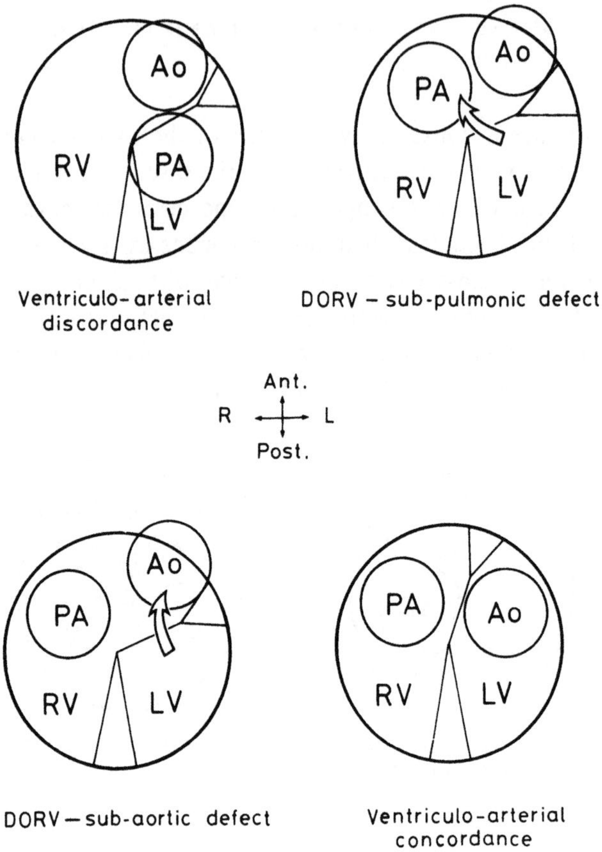

Figure 14. Diagram illustrating how a comparable spectrum to that illustrated in Figure 13 can exist when the *pulmonary artery* is 'plugged' into the posterior outflow tract. Anatomical evidence substantiates the existence of this spectrum (See references 43-46).

known that specimens exist which demonstrate the presence of a similar spectrum except for the aorta being left-sided rather than right-sided (fig. 14). Thus hearts exist in which the aorta arises anteriorly from the left ventricle in left sided position. These can exist with or without aortic-mitral continuity (42, 43). There is a transition from these hearts to double outlet right ventricle with sub-aortic defect and left sided aorta (44). It is known that double outlet right ventricle with left sided aorta can exhibit exactly the same variability as double outlet right ventricle with right sided aorta (45). Finally, specimens have been described which illustrate the transition from double outlet right ventricle with sub-pulmonary defect and left sided aorta to ventriculo-arterial discordance with left sided aorta (46). Thus two spectra exist which from the standpoint of infundibular malformation are very similar. The difference between them is that in one the aorta is a left sided structure whereas in the other it is right sided. (Compare Figures 13 and 14). It seems reasonable to suggest that the link between the two is the mode of septation of the truncus. Both are dependent upon infundibular maldevelopment to produce the transition from anomaly. However, the change between the two spectra is likely to be produced by the 'plugging-in' of the aortic sac to the bulbus, however this is accomplished. Evidence from malformed hearts therefore indicates most strongly that both infundibular maldevelopment and truncal malseptation can themselves produce ventriculo-arterial discordance, but that both are required to co-exist so as to explain the full range of infundibulo-truncal malformations.

SUMMARY

It has been indicated that many of the arguments concerning transposition result from its definition either as a relation or a connexion. To avoid such controversy, the malformation presently discussed has been defined as ventriculo-arterial discordance, being the situation in which the aorta arises from the morphologically right ventricle and the pulmonary artery from the morphologically left ventricle. Two basic concepts have previously been advanced to account for the genesis of this anomaly; the one pointing to infundibular maldevelopment and the other to truncal malseptation. Normal development relevant to this concept is briefly reviewed. It is then suggested that this information, together with evidence from malformed hearts, indicates that both hypotheses can account for ventriculo-arterial discordance. Indeed it is likely that the two must co-exist to produce the full range of known infundibulo-truncal malformations.

REFERENCES

1. Kirklin, J. W., Pacifico, A. D., Bargeron, L. M. Jr., Soto, B., Cardiac repair in anatomically corrected malposition of the great arteries. *Circulation* 48, 153 (1973).
2. de la Cruz, M. V., Amoedo, M., Rivera, F. and Attie, F., Atrioventricular relations and their classification. Two specimens of arterioventricular discordance and review of published reports. *Br. Heart J.* 36, 539 (1974).
3. Keith, A., Malformations of the bulbus cordis. An unrecognised division of the human heart. In: Bullock, E. H. (ed.) *Studies in Pathology*. Aberdeen, 1906.

4. Keith, A., Hunterian lectures on malformations of the heart. *Lancet 2*, 433 (1909).
5. Keith, A., Fate of the bulbus cordis in the human heart. *Lancet 2*, 1267 (1924).
6. Lev, M. and Saphir, O., Transposition of the large vessels. *J. Tech. Methods* 17, 126 (1937).
7. Harris, J. S. and Farber, S., Transposition of the great cardiac vessels with special reference to the phylogenetic theory of Spitzer. *Arch. Pathol.* 28, 427 (1939).
8. Spitzer, A., *Handbuch der speziellen pathologischen Anatomie und Histologie*. Berlin, 1924.
9. Rokitansky, C. von, *Die Defekte der Scheidewände des Herzens*. Braumüller, Vienna, 1875.
10. de la Cruz, M. V. and da Rocha, J. P., An ontogenetic theory for the explanation of congenital malformations involving the truncus and conus. *Am. Heart J.* 51, 782 (1956).
11. Van Mierop, L. H. S., Alley, R. D., Kausel, H. W. and Stranahan, A., Pathogenesis of transposition complexes. I. Embryology of the ventricles and great arteries. *Am. J. Cardiol.* 12, 216 (1963a).
12. Van Mierop, L. H. S. and Wiglesworth, F. W., Pathogenesis of transposition complexes. II. Anomalies due to faulty transfer of the posterior great artery. *Am. J. Cardiol.* 12, 226 (1963b).
13. Van Mierop, L. H. S. and Wiglesworth, F. W., Pathogenesis of transposition complexes. III. True transposition of the great vessels. *Am. J. Cardiol.* 12, 233 (1963c).
14. Van Praagh, R., Ongley, P. A. and Swan, J. C., Anatomic types of single or common ventricle in man. *Am. J. Cardiol.* 13, 367 (1964).
15. Van Praagh, R. and Van Praagh, S., Isolated ventricular inversion. A consideration of the morphogenesis and diagnosis of transposed and non-transposed great arteries. *Am. J. Cardiol.* 17, 395 (1966).
16. Paul, M. H., Van Praagh, S. and Van Praagh, R., Transposition of the great arteries. In: Watson, H. (ed.) *Paediatric Cardiology*, London 1968.
17. Van Praagh, R., Perez-Trevino, C., Lopez-Cuellar, M., Baker, F. W., Zuberbuhler, J. R., Quero, M., Perez, V. M., Moreno, F., Van Praagh, S., Transposition of the great arteries with posterior aorta, anterior pulmonary artery, subpulmonary conus and fibrous continuity between aortic and atrioventricular valves. *Am. J. Cardiol.* 28, 621 (1971).
18. Van Praagh, R., The segmental approach to diagnosis in congenital heart disease. In: *Birth Defects: Original Article Series* 8, No. 4. Baltimore 1972.
19. Van Praagh. R. Conotruncus malformations. In: *Heart Disease in Infancy – Diagnosis and Surgical Treatment*, p. 86. Ed. by B. G. Barrett-Boyas, J. M. Neutze and E. A. Harris. Churchill Livingstone, Edinburgh.
20. Butler, J. K., *An experimental analysis of cardiac loop formation in the chick*. M.A. Thesis, University of Texas, 1952.
21. Pernkopf, E. and Wirtinger, W., Die Transposition der Herzostien, ein Versuch der Erklärung dieser Erscheinung. *Z. Anat. Entwickl. gesch.* 100, 563 (1933).
22. Asami, I., Beitrag zur Entwicklung des Kammerseptums im menschlichen Herzen mit besonderer Berücksichtigung der sogenannten Bulbusdrehung. *Z. Anat. Entwickl. gesch.* 128, 1 (1969).
23. Goor, D. A., Dische, R. and Lillehei, C. W., The conotruncus. I. Its normal inversion and conus absorption. *Circulation* 46, 375 (1972).
24. Goor, D. A. and Edwards, J. E., The spectrum of transposition of the great arteries: with specific reference to developmental anatomy of the conus. *Circulation* 48, 406 (1973).
25. Lev, M., Bharati, S., Meng, C. C. L., Liberthson, R. R., Paul, M. H. and Idriss, F., A concept of double outlet right ventricle. *J. Thorac. Cardiovasc. Surg.* 64, 271 (1972).
26. Lev. M. and Eckner, F. A. O., Embryologic, pathogenetic and pathologic considerations. In: *Heart Disease in Children.* Gasul, B. M., Arcilla, R. A. and Lev, M., Philadelphia 1966. p. 21.
27. Anderson, R. H., Wilkinson, J. L., Arnold, R. and Lubkiewicz, K., Morphogenesis of bulboventricular malformations. I. Consideration of embryogenesis in the normal heart. *Br. Heart J.* 36, 242 (1974a).

28. Anderson, R. H., Wilkinson, J. L., Arnold, R., Becker, A. E. and Lubkiewicz, K., Morphogenesis of bulboventricular malformations. II. Observations on malformed hearts. *Br. Heart J.* 36, 948 (1974b).
29. Quero- Jimenez, M. and Perez Martinez, V., Uncommon conal pathology in complete dextroposition of the great arteries with ventricular septal defect. *Chest* 66, 411 (1974).
30. Thiene, G., Razzolini, R. and Dalla-Volta, S., Aorto-pulmonary relationship, arterio-ventricular alignment and ventricular septal defects in complete transposition of the great arteries. *Eur. J. Cardiol.* 4, 13 (1976).
31. Doerr, W., Zur Transposition der Herzschlagadern (Ein kritischer Beitrag zur Lehre der Transposition) *Virchows Arch. (path. Anat.)* 303, 168 (1938).
32. Doerr, W., Die formale Entstehung der wichtigsten Missbildungen des arteriellen Herzendes. *Beitr. pathol. Anat.* 115, 1 (1955).
33. Doerr, W., Die Missbildungen des Herzens und der grossen Gefässe. In: Kaufmann, E. and Staemmler, M. (ed.) *Lehrbuch der speziellen pathologischen Anatomie*, Berlin 1955.
34. Bersch, W., On the importance of the bulboauricular flange for the formal genesis of congenital heart defects with special regard to the ventricular septum defects. *Virchows Arch. Abt. A.* 354, 252 (1971).
35. Chuaqui, B. and Bersch, W., The formal genesis of the transposition of the great arteries. *Virchows Arch. Abt. A. Path. Anat.* 358, 11 (1973).
36. Goerttler, K., Die Stoffwechseltopographie des embryonalen Hühnchenherzens und ihre Bedeutung für die Entstehung angeborener Herzfehlern. *Verh. Dtsch. Ges. Pathol.* 40, 181 (1956).
37. Los, J. A., Embryology. In: Watson, H. (ed.) *Paediatric Cardiology*. London 1968.
38. Van Mierop, L. H. S. and Gessner, I. H., Pathogenetic mechanisms in congenital cardiovascular malformations. *Prog. Cardiovasc. Dis.* 15, 67 (1972).
39. Carr, I., Tynan, M., Aberdeen, E., Bonham-Carter, R. E., Grahan, G. and Waterston, D. J., Predictive accuracy of the 'loop rule' in 109 children with classical complete transposition of the great arteries (T.G.A.) (abstr.) *Circulation* 38, suppl. VI-52 (1968).
40. Lincoln, J. C. R., Hasse, J., Anderson, R. H. and Shinebourne, E. A., Surgical correction in complete levotransposition of the great arteries with an unusual subaortic ventricular septal defect. *Am. J. Cardiol.* 38, 344 (1976).
41. Los, J. A., Een eenvoudig ruimtelijk schema voor het classificeren van stoornissen in het septeringsproces van het menselijke hart naar morfogenetische criteria. *Ned. Tijdschr. Geneesk.* 120, 100 (1976).
42. Quero-Jimenez, M. and Raposo-Sonnenfeld, I., Isolated ventricular inversion with situs solitus. *Br. Heart J.* 37, 293 (1975).
43. Anderson, R. H., Becker, A. E., Losekoot, T. G. and Gerlis, L. M., Anatomically corrected malposition of great arteries. *Br. Heart J.* 37, 993 (1975).
44. Lincoln, J. C. R., Anderson, R. H., Shinebourne, E. A., English, T. A. H. and Wilkinson, J. L., Double outlet right ventricle with l-malposition of the aorta. *Br. Heart J.* 37, 453 (1975).
45. Anderson, R. H., Pickering, D. and Brown, R., Double outlet right ventricle with l-malposition and uncommitted ventricular septal defect. *Eur. J. Cardiol.* 3, 133 (1975).
46. Shafer, A. B., Lopez, J. F., Kline, I. K. and Lev, M., Truncal inversion with biventricular pulmonary trunk and aorta from right ventricle (variant of Taussig-Bing complex) *Circulation* 36, 383 (1967).

11. THE FORMAL MORPHOGENESIS OF ARTERIAL TRANSPOSITION WITH SPECIAL REGARD TO THE CONCEPT OF HOMOLOGY AND SERIES FORMATION

W. BERSCH

For more than a century now the malformation of the arterial end of the heart and the arterial transposition in particular have caused anatomists and pathologists alike to draw up classifications and concepts pertaining to the genesis of these cardiac malformations.

A decisive change in the often rather controversial views on this malformations problem was brought about by the discussion of Spitzer's phylogenetic theory (1, 2, 3) and the ontogenetic interpretation of Pernkopf and Wirtinger (4, 5) by Doerr (6-9) and his resulting concept of the formal principle of 'vectorial bulbus rotation' (10-15) in normal cardiogenesis in the sense of an embryologico-evolutionary series (16).

According to this principle the malformations – the Eisenmenger complex, the tetralogy of Fallot, the Taussig-Bing anomaly and the crossed transposition – can be understood as a uniform process in a teratologic series, i.e. they can be explained by the extent of the arrest of the vectorial rotation of the bulbus.

To facilitate a general view of this paper the topics will be arranged in the following order:

1. A few remarks on the significance of the concept of homology and of the embryologico-teratologic series as a model-oriented morphological working method in pathology.
2. Some problems relating to the morphogenesis of congenital heart defects which will involve a discussion of the principle of vectorial bulbus rotation.
3. An attempt to eliminate so far as possible conceivable contradictions to other theories on the genesis of the transposition.
4. General conceptual criteria relating to the nature of the arterial transposition.

1. HOMOLOGY AND EMBRYOLOGICO-TERATOLOGIC SERIES, A MODEL-ORIENTED WORKING METHOD

The methodical concepts of homology and series and inextricably connected with them the construction of models, have been familiar to biologists and physicians since about the 17th century.

In probably all fields of science, the methodical application of models for systematic investigation of special problems is a generally used method of scientific research whenever a process is not open to 'immediate intuition'.

With his primeval plant Goethe created a model of a special nature. He thus became the founder of so-called idealistic morphology and typology, which is difficult to understand without knowing Plato's theory of ideas, but allows for great intellectual flexibility and became the basis of the comparative method later applied by Geoffroy de St. Hilaire in classical morphology.

This method, actually established by Geoffroy de St. Hilaire and strictly speaking set up by Goethe, became after Owen (17) had formed the concept of 'homology' later so to speak the property of comparative anatomy and remained controversial for a long time.

The establishment of homology is an intellectual model of comparative intuition providing uniform images for a plurality of things and thus has a purely formal and thus absolute character.

However, the concept of homology finds a practical application in studies of morphological series, the great heuristic significance of which for pathology seems to have been recognized first by Schwalbe (16). With regard to the theory of malformations we have thus at the one end of the morphologico-teratologic series the normal finding or only a slight deviation from it (late teratologic point of determination) while there is a high degree of malformation at the other end (early teratologic point of determination). Thus studies of critically examined series may in the first place be based on a classification principle with the objective of creating the best possible general view of the phenomena under consideration, the general aim being to infer the existence of a fundamental process from the repetition of stereotype features! However, it must always be born in mind that in the sense of Goethe's typology only formal but not causal relations can be stated: 'What is equal as regards form can be different as regards its nature' (18).

The situation may be summarized as follows: 'the concept of homology and its practical application in the study of morphological series as a model-oriented method of morphology – morphology still being a fundamental method of pathology'.

2. VECTORIAL BULBUS ROTATION

A survey of cardiac development in the course of time shows that the decisive events take place between the 10th and 48th day of embryonic development. The greatest frequency of events, according to Streeter's horizons, is found between the XIIIth and XXth horizons (19), i.e. between the 28th and 41th day of the ovulation age. During this period three essential processes take place, which of course, go 'hand in hand' but will be dealt with separately for didactic reasons.

1. The right section of the auricular canal, which at the moment of the cardiac loop is connected only to the proampulla, due to its medial and dorsal displacement and a 90 degree clockwise rotation about its own axis gains connection with the enlarging metampulla (vectorial rotation of the auricular canal (20, 21)).

2. At the arterial end of the heart a complex process of movements occurs as a result of three components (fig. 1):

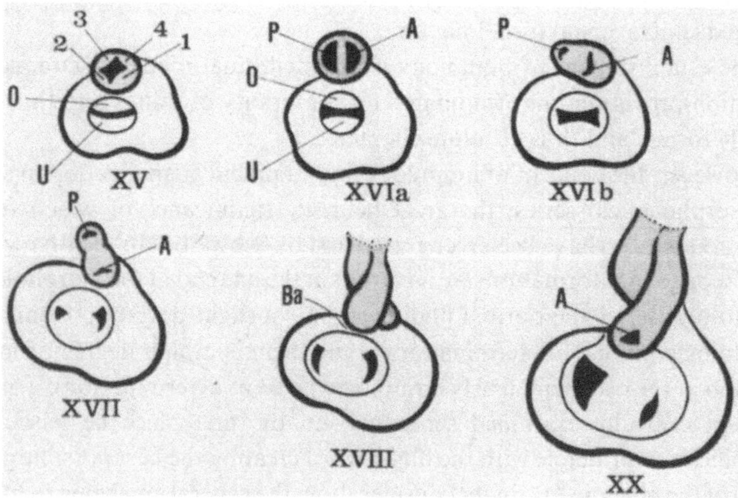

Figure 1. Schematic representation of the stages of the bulbotruncal torsion in the heart of a human embryo. Top view (atria removed). At top ventral, at bottom dorsal. The Roman numerals designate the developmental stages. 1, 2, 3 and 4 = distal bulbar swellings; P = pulmonary orifice; A = aortic orifice. From stage XV to stage XVII a rotation of the bulbotruncal orifice and the arterial orifices respectively can be seen (vectorial bulbar torsion). In stage XVIII the bulboauricular flange (Ba) is still visible. Final position of the aortic orifice after recession of the bulboauricular flange (Ba) in stage XX. O = anterior, U = posterior principal endocardial cushion. Schematical and changed according to the original photograms by Asami 1969 (from Bersch and Doerr, Reitende Gefässe des Herzens, Springer Verlag, 1976).

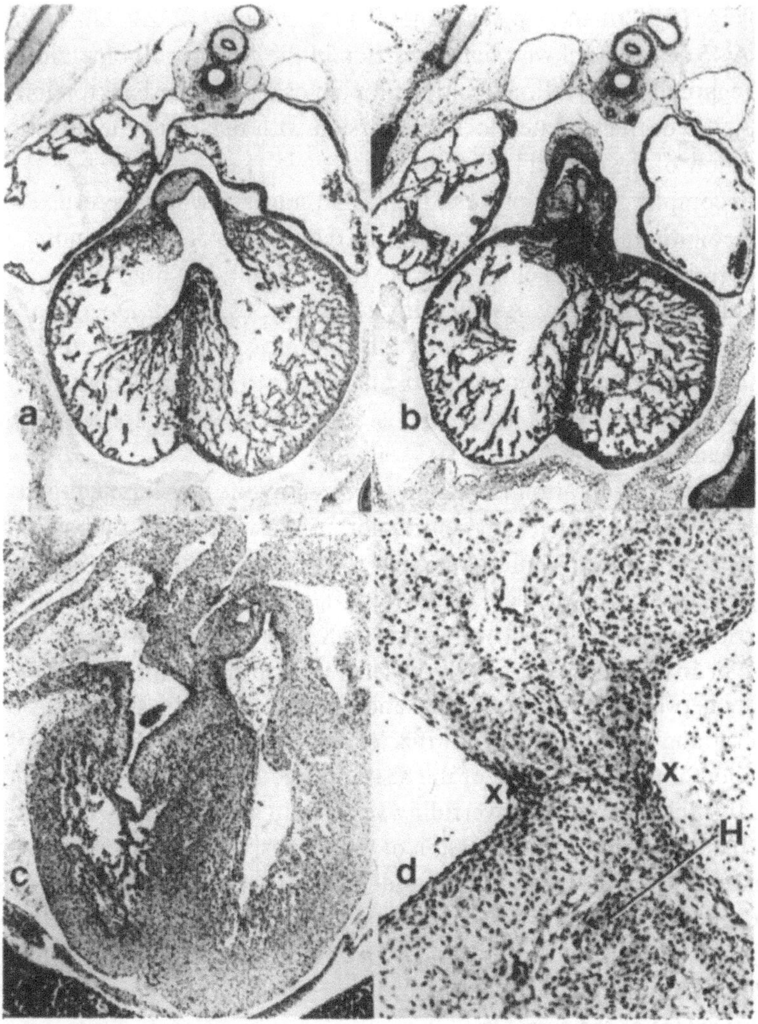

Figure 2a-d. Synopsis of the decisive steps of the complex successive events of the vectorial bulbar torsion according to the principle of a 'embryological-evolutionary' series. Frontal views of human embryonal hearts at evolutionary stage XVIII (a and b) and XIX (c and d). *a:* 'riding' aorta over the foramen interventriculare still open. *b:* evident shrinkage of the bulbus with nearly straight bulbar ridges, which have united towards the bulbar septum (first component of the vectorial bulbar torsion). *c:* the foramen interventriculare is completely closed and the aortic ostium has gained connexion with the left ventricle. *d:* clearly visible 'sutureline' (x-x) between the principal ridge and the counter ridge. Beneath the principal ridge first structural elements of His' bundle (H). Modified after Bersch and Doerr, 1976.

a. A leftward displacement of the entire bulbus together with a bulbar shrinkage (fig. 2b) and a displacement of the truncus (22, 23, 24).

b. A 45 degree clockwise bulbar torsion of the ostium bulbometampullare with regard to the direction of blood flow (so-called 'bulbar backtorsion' (4)).

c. A 150 degree counterclockwise torsion with regard to the direction of blood flow of the ostium bulbotruncale.

This complex rotation process, the partial stages of which were also found by other authors (23, 24), has been verified by means of corresponding findings of serial sections of embryonic hearts (25, 26). It has been stereomicroscopically confirmed by Asami's investigations (22) and Doerr called it 'vectorial bulbar torsion' as a 'unity' of a plurality of events. 'Vector' means that the arterial outlet – bulbus and truncus have to be regarded as a uniform entity – migrates over a field, and is at the same time exposed to other movements.

3. Ventricular septation is basically realized by the development and subsequent fusion of the septum ventriculorum musculare, the bulbar septum and the counter-ridge ('bulbo-auricular ridge' (27)), with the aorta still overriding the open interventricular foramen (fig. 2a) during the XVIII. horizon ('overriding aorta', (23, 24)), in stage XIX (fig. 2c) the aortic ostium has gained definitive connection with the left ventricle and a suture-line (fig. 2d) appears between the principal ridge and the counter-ridge (28).

Everything that might disturb this 'evolutionary series' (fig. 2a-d) of the formation of the normal end of the heart (= vectorial bulbar torsion) could cause the phenomenon of 'overriding vessels'. In general it may be said that disturbances of the vectorial torsion of the bulbus, formally due to a varying extent of arrest of the torsion, will result in heterotopies of the great vessels at the arterial end of the heart, the individual forms of which constitute a 'teratologic series' found by Doerr (10-15). According to this the following separately occurring malformations can be explained depending on the respective extent of the arrest (fig. 3):

The greatest arrest (the 'one' end of the series and at the same time the earliest point of determination) is shown in the origin of both arterial trunks from the so-called 'right ventricle' (double outlet right ventricle, usually, but not always in 'transposed position' as a sign of the arrest of the bulbotruncal torsion. The mildest form of the arrest of the torsion (the 'other' end of the series and at the same time the least deviation from the normal position) is represented by the overriding aorta in the Eisenmenger complex.

In between, depending on the respective extent of the arrest, there are the crossed transposition with the 'leading phenomenon' of the 'absence of twist-

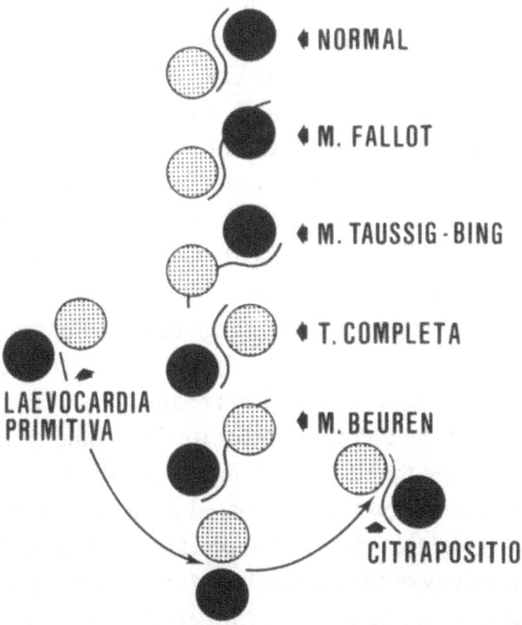

Figure 3. Schematic representation of a 'teratologic series' of the heterotopies of the great vessels at the arterial end of the heart, formally due to an arrest of the vectorial bulbar torsion. Top view of the arterial orifices. Black = aortic orifice; dotted = pulmonary orifice; S-shaped line = ventricular septum. Left: primitive stage before the beginning of the vectorial bulbar torsion. Between these stages in the direction of the arrow towards the position at the lower centre we have all transitional stages of so-called primitive levocardia ('double outlet right ventricle'). An anomalous displacement (direction of arrow on the right side of the picture) will result in a citraposition = corrected transposition. The Eisenmenger complex would have to be placed between Morbus Fallot and the normal position (top centre of picture). (From Bersch and Doerr, Reitende Gefässe des Herzens, Springer-Verlag, 1976.)

ing' of the great vessels, i.e. the parallel upward position with straight septum (disturbance or arrest of the bulbotruncal torsion), the Beuren anomaly with overriding pulmonary artery (dorsally), the Taussig-Bing anomaly with the aorta in righthand dorsal position and the pulmonary artery in lefthand ventral position and finally the tetralogy of Fallot with overriding aorta.

3. COMPATIBILITY WITH OTHER THEORIES

The decisive factors giving rise to the term 'vectorial bulbar torsion' have been described. Depending on the point of determination, a disturbance of any kind in this process may result in one or other malformation of the arterial outflow tracts as part of the malformation series described, of which the crossed arterial transposition is a part. The nature of this disturbance, however, remained uncertain until Shaner (29, 30), who examined many thousands of hearts of embryo pigs, became the first to point out the significance of a collision of the dorsal circumference of the aortic orifice with the anterior luxuriantly structured auricular endocardial cushion which has not receded in time. This resulted in an emphasis on the importance of both growth and cellular decay in embryonic development (31), without which the enormous movement of material for the purpose of a differentiating development would be inconceivable. Varying growth activities of the embryonic myocardium could be experimentally verified (32, 33) and cardiac malformations corresponding to disturbances in the formal change of the arterial end of the heart in the course of the vectorial bulbar torsion, could be produced experimentally by inhibiting the zones with active growth (34).

Grant's (35) transposition theory is based on such growth differences. In the otherwise turbulent cardiac development, he assumes a fibrous continuum at the concavity of the cardiac loop (the later heart skeleton) to be a fixed point, which by an anomalous shift to the left, would result in the transposition of the vessels. From this he derives the absence of the fibrous continuity between aortic and mitral valves (regio mitroaortique) as the leading symptom.

Richard and Stella Van Praagh and their colleagues (36-39) have also based their theory on growth considerations. With reference to Keith's theory of bulbar atrophy (40), they explain all formal anomalies that can be derived from an anomalous connection of the aortic and pulmonary arteries to the ventricular base by a growth disturbance of the bulbus, which they call conus. This so-called conal growth hypothesis has met with general approval. Goor and his colleagues (23), however, do not agree completely! While demonstrating a shrinkage of the conus, they afterwards expressly speak of free torsions (leftward shift of the ostium bulbi), which would occur before conal development!

Van Praagh's study group (39), moreover, tends to give the word 'transposition' an apparently new definition in the sense of 'dislocation', and raises the question whether it would not be better to speak of a 'malposition', which in turn, has not remained uncontradicted (41).

To summarize we might characterize the situation in the following way: no cardiac differentiation without growth, no movement of material without decay and addition of cells; but also no doubt that there are free complex motion processes in the definitive formal change of the embryonic heart.

The conal growth hypothesis is thus characterized as a programme, it is an important element of biotechnics, i.e. of the mechanism of definitive formation, and thus it is in no way incompatible with the formal concept of vectorial bulbar torsion.

4. CRITERIA RELATING TO THE NATURE OF TRANSPOSITION

No one has so far seen an embryonic human heart during the transposition, nor has anyone identified a heart during this process (19, Anderson, this book, page 93), on the other hand, during the process of cardiac development – almost as a short-lived transitory stage of a biologically continuous process – there will 'normally' occur a transpositional arrangement of the great vessels.

As a consequence, there is no major difficulty in explaining the conventional transpositions, in agreement with the different concepts – in the sense of a 'field of factors' –, in a formally morphogenetic way as a result of the disturbance of the complex rotation and growth processes.

Which anomaly is to be considered the criterion, i.e. the essential morphological symptom in the definitive cardiac malformation of the 'crossed arterial transposition', depends on the author's view of the genesis. Grant and Van Praagh have derived the mitroaortic discontinuity as a symptom. Cases of crossed transposition and a fibrous mitroaortic continuity over a VSD thus actually could not be regarded as transpositions (42).

On the other hand, the concept which considers an arrest of the bulbotruncal torsion – in the sense of an inhibitive malformation (16) – to be the morpho-pathogenetic principle of arterial transposition (19, 43), regards the parallel position of the great arteries, i.e. the absence of twisting as the 'leading phenomenon'.

Thus transposition will occur frequently but not necessarily in the absence of the septum ventriculorum or in cases of 'double outlet right ventricle' (44, 45). This shows that the use of this morphological phenomenon as a diagnostic criterion will allow for an improved typology of apparently very different types of malformation and thus for a simplified principle of classification. Finally, it should be emphasized that – as Doerr (6, 8, 46) has already pointed out – the inversion, which occurs in the morphological cycle of the arterial transposition in the form of the so-called corrected transposition, is to be regarded as a phenomenon that is formally not related to the transposition (47). The corrected transposition is consequently not a special form of the arterial transposition but, in agreement with De la Cruz et al. (48) a ventricular inversion with transpositional arrangement of the great vessels.

However, in view of the nature of the phenomena, it will always remain difficult to find neatly separated morphological entities within a biological continuum. A major step towards simplification seems to be the methodical principle of studying critically examined morphological-teratologic series as discussed in the introduction of this paper.

REFERENCES

1. Spitzer, A., Über die Ursachen und Mechanismen der Zweiteilung des Wirbeltierherzens. *Wilhelm Roux' Arch. Entwickl. mech. Org.* 45, 686 (1919).
2. Spitzer, A., Über den Bauplan des normalen und missgebildeten Herzens. Versuch einer phylogenetischen Theorie. *Virchows Arch. pathol. Anat.* 243, 81 (1923).
3. Spitzer, A., Über Dextroversion, Transposition und Inversion des Herzens und die gegenseitige Larvierung der beiden letzten Anomalien, nebst Bemerkungen über das Wesen des Situs Inversus. *Virchows Arch. pathol. Anat.* 271, 226 (1929).
4. Pernkopf, E. & Wirtinger, W., Die Transposition der Herzostien, ein Versuch der Erklärung dieser Erscheinung. I: Die Phoronomie der Herzentwicklung als morphogenetische Grundlage der Erklärung. *Z. Anat. Entwickl. gesch.* 100, 561 (1933).
5. Pernkopf, E. & Wirtinger, W., Das Wesen der Transposition im Gebiet des Herzens, ein Versuch der Erklärung auf entwicklungsgeschichtlicher Grundlage. *Virchows Arch. pathol. Anat.* 295, 143 (1935).
6. Doerr, W., Zwei weitere Fälle von Herzmissbildungen. Ein Beitrag zu Spitzer's phylogenetischer Theorie. *Virchows Arch. pathol. Anat.* 301, 668 (1938).
7. Doerr, W., Zur Transposition der Herzschlagadern. Ein kritischer Beitrag zur Lehre der Transpositionen. *Virchows Arch. pathol. Anat.* 303, 168 (1938/39).
8. Doerr, W., Über Missbildungen des menschlichen Herzens mit besonderer Berücksichtigung von Bulbus und Trunkus. *Virchows Arch. pathol. Anat.* 310, 304 (1943).
9. Doerr, W., Morphogenese und Korrelation chirurgisch wichtiger angeborener Herzfehler. *Ergebn. Chir. Orthop.* 36, 1 (1950).
10. Doerr, W., Pathologische Anatomie typischer Grundformen angeborener Herzfehler. *Monatsschr. Kinderheilk.* 100, 107 (1952a).
11. Doerr, W., Über ein formales Prinzip der Koppelung von Entwicklungsstörungen der venösen und arteriellen Kammerostien. *Z. Kreisl. forsch.* 41, 269 (1952b).
12. Doerr, W., Die formale Entstehung der wichtigsten Missbildungen des arteriellen Herzendes. *Beitr. pathol. Anat.* 115, 1 (1955a).
13. Doerr, W., Missbildungen des Herzens und der grossen Gefässe. In: Kaufmann, E. & Staemmler, M. (eds.), *Lehrbuch der speziellen pathologischen Anatomie*, Bd. I/1, Berlin 1955.
14. Doerr, W., Pathologische Anatomie der angeborenen Herzfehler. In: von Bergmann, G., Frey, W. & Schwiegk, H. (eds.), *Handbuch der Inneren Medizin*, 4. Aufl. Bd. IX, 3, 1, Berlin 1960.
15. Doerr, W., Allgemeine Pathologie der Organe des Kreislaufs. In: Meessen, H. & Roulet, F. (eds.), *Handbuch der allgemeinen Pathologie*, Bd. III/4, Berlin 1970.
16. Schwalbe, E., *Die Morphologie der Misbildungen des Menschen und der Tiere* I: Allgemeine Missbildungslehre (Teratologie), Jena 1906.
17. Owen, R., On the archetype and homologies of the vertebrate skeleton. *Report 16th Meeting Br. Ass. Adv. Sc.*, London 1848.

18. Letterer, E., *Allgemeine Pathologie, Grundlagen und Probleme*, Stuttgart 1959.
19. Bersch, W. & Doerr, W., Reitende Gefässe des Herzens. Homologiebegriff und Reihenbildung. In: *Sitzungsberichte der Heidelberger Akademie der Wissenschaften*, mathematisch-naturwissenschaftliche Klasse 1, Heidelberg 1976.
20. Goerttler, K., *Normale und pathologische Entwicklung des menschlichen Herzens*. Zwanglose Abhandl. aus dem Gebiet der normalen und pathol. Anat., Heft 3, Stuttgart 1958.
21. Goerttler, K., Entwicklungsgeschichte des Herzens. In: Bargmann, W. & Doerr, W. (eds.), *Das Herz des Menschen*, Bd. I, Stuttgart 1963.
22. Asami, I., Beitrag zur Entwicklung des Kammerseptums im menschlichen Herzen mit besonderer Berücksichtigung der sog. Bulbusdrehung. *Z. Anat. Entwickl. gesch.* 128, 1 (1969).
23. Goor, D. A., Dische, R. & Lillehei, W., The conotruncus. I. Its normal inversion and conus absorption. *Circulation* 46, 375 (1972).
24. Anderson, R. H., Wilkinson, J. L., Arnold, R. & Lubkiewicz, K., Morphogenesis of bulboventricular malformations I: Consideration of embryogenesis in the normal heart. *Br. Heart J.* 36, 242 (1974).
25. Chuaqui, J. B. & Bersch, W., The periods of determination of cardiac malformations. *Virchows Arch. Abt. A.* 356, 95 (1972).
26. Chuaqui, J. B. & Bersch, W., The formal genesis of the transposition of the great arteries. *Virchows Arch. Abt. A.* 358, 11 (1973).
27. Bersch, W., On the importance of the bulboauricular flange for the formal genesis of congenital heart defects with special regard to the ventricular septum defects. *Virchows Arch. Abt. A.* 354, 252 (1971).
28. Bersch., W., Über das Moderatorband der linken Herzkammer. *Basic Res. Cardiol.* 68, 225 (1973).
29. Shaner, R. F., Malformation of the atrioventricular endocardial cushion of the embryo pig and its relation to defects of the conus and truncus arteriosus. *Am. J. Anat.* 84, 431 (1949).
30. Shaner, R. F., Complete and corrected transposition of the aorta, pulmonary artery and ventricles in pig embryos, and a case of corrected transposition in a child. *Am. J. Anat.* 88, 35 (1951).
31. Pexieder, T., Cell death in the morphogenesis and teratogenesis of the heart. *Adv. Anat. Embryol. Cell Biol.* vol. 51/3, Berlin 1975.
32. Goerttler, K., Stoffwechseltopographie des embryonalen Hühnchenherzens und ihre Bedeutung für die Entstehung angeborener Herzfehler. *Verh. Dtsch. Ges. Path.* 40, 181 (1956).
33. Grohmann, D., Mitotische Wachstumsaktivität des embryonalen und fetalen Hühnchenherzens und ihre Bedeutung für die Entstehung von Herzmissbildungen. *Z. Zellforsch.* 55, 104 (1961).
34. Wegener, K., Über die experimentelle Erzeugung von Herzmissbildungen durch Trypanblau. *Arch. Kreisl. forsch.* 34, 99 (1961).
35. Grant, R. P., Morphogenesis of transposition of the great vessels. *Circulation* 26, 819 (1962).
36. Van Praagh, R. & Van Praagh, S., Isolated ventricular inversion. A consideration of the morphogenesis, definition and diagnosis of non-transposed and transposed great arteries. *Am. J. Cardiol.* 17, 395 (1966).
37. Van Praagh, R., Anatomically corrected transposition of the great arteries. *Br. Heart J.* 29, 112 (1967).
38. Van Praagh, R., Vlad, P. & Keith, J. D., Complete transposition of the great arteries. In: Keith, J. D., Rowe, R. D. & Vlad, P., *Heart disease in infancy and childhood*, 2nd ed., New York 1967.
39. Van Praagh, R., Pèrez-Trevino, C., Lopez-Cuellar, M. et al., Transposition of the great arteries with posterior aorta, anterior pulmonary artery, subpulmonary conus and fibrous continuity between aortic and atrioventricular valves. *Am. J. Cardiol.* 28, 621 (1971).

40. Keith, A., The Hunterian lectures on malformations of the heart. Lecture II. *Lancet*, 433 (1909, II).
41. Van Mierop, L. H. S., Transposition of the great arteries. I. Clarification or further confusion? *Am. J. Cardiol.* 28, 735 (1971).
42. Van Praagh, R., Transposition of the great arteries. II. Transposition clarified. *Am. J. Cardiol.* 28, 739 (1971).
43. Bersch, W., Chuaqui, J. B. & Heilmann, K., Persistenz des primitiven Aortenconus bei regelrechter Stellung der grossen Gefässe des Herzens. *Virchows Arch. [Pathol. Anat.]* 368, 299 (1975).
44a. Van Mierop, L. H. S. & Wiglesworth, F. W., Pathogenesis of transposition complexes II. Anomalies due to faulty transfer of the posterior great artery. *Am. J. Cardiol.* 12, 226 (1963a).
44b. Van Mierop, L. H. S. & Wiglesworth, F. W., Pathogenesis of transposition complexes III. True transposition of the great vessels. *Am. J. Cardiol.* 12, 233 (1963b).
45. Goor, D. A. & Edwards, J. E., The conotruncus II. Report of a case showing persistent aortic conus and lack of inversion of the truncus (a bulboventricular heart). *Circulation* 46, 385 (1972).
46. Doerr, W., Über den Situs inversus im Gebiet des Herzens. *Dtsch. Med. Wochenschr.* 72, 570 (1947).
47. Chuaqui, J. B., Zur Terminologie einiger Herzheterotopien. *Virchows Arch. Abt. A.* 347, 260 (1969).
48. De la Cruz, M. V., Espino-Vela, J., Attie, F. & Munoz, L., An embryological theory for the ventricular inversions and their classification. *Am. Heart J.* 73, 777 (1967).

12. TRANSPOSITION OF THE GREAT ARTERIES: CONTROVERSIES CONCERNING THE NATURE AND THE PATHOGENESIS OF THE ANOMALY

L. H. S. VAN MIEROP

In many ways transposition of the great arteries (TGA) continues to be somewhat of an enigma. No cardiovascular anomaly has received more attention and generated more discussion and controversy for as long a time. Even the validity of its name has recently been questioned (1) and no one as yet has been able to define it to everyone's satisfaction. Not surprisingly, therefore, there continues to be disagreement among 'experts' concerning its pathogenesis.

By correlating observations made on malformed hearts and those made on normal hearts and the developing cardiovascular system, it is often possible to arrive at a reasonably plausible explanation as to what might have happened pathogenetically in the case of a particular cardiac anomaly. This approach, however, does not work very well in the case of transposition of the great arteries – at least it hasn't for me. Over the past 20 years I have studied hundreds of serially sectioned embryos of various ages and of a number of mammalian species, and I have made wax plate reconstructions of many of their hearts. Yet I have not been able to find a stage of development in which the embryonic heart resembles the great artery-ventricular relationships seen in transposition of the great arteries.

The term 'transposition of the great arteries' appears to have been used first by Farre in 1814 (2). The title of the particular section of his monograph in which he described the cardiac malformation was 'Transposition of the Aorta and Pulmonary Artery'. Farre first refers to a heart described previously in 1789 by M. Baillie, whom he quotes verbatim, stating that 'the aorta arose out of the right ventricle, and the pulmonary artery out of the left.' He then mentions a similar case reported by a Mr. Langstaff. In describing the third case Farre used the term 'transposition of the great arteries' on two occasions, but did not define it. On page 30 of his paper there is an interesting and, I think, very important passage if we are going to try to guess as to what he had in mind when he used the term 'transposition'. The first paragraph on page 30 reads as follows: 'The ventricles altered in their figure; but some allowance must be made for their structure. The ventricles themselves can be said to be transposed only in respect to their figure, in the relative thickness of their walls; for the right valve is tricuspidal and the left mitral. It seems unnecessary to add another figure to illustrate these facts.' Here, therefore, Farre used the term 'transposition' in reference to the ventricles. Apparently he asked himself whether, in the specimen, not only the arteries but also the ventricles might possibly be transposed (i.e. reversed in their relative positions), and dismissed this possibility on the grounds that the right A-V valve was a tricuspid valve and the left A-V valve a mitral. Farre apparently used the term 'transposition' in the usual sense (i.e., two structures or entities have taken up each other's position).

Since all three hearts represented cases of uncomplicated transposition of the great arteries, *any such exchange in position of the two great arteries in an otherwise normal heart, of necessity, will result in the aorta arising anteriorly from the right ventricle, while the pulmonary trunk will occupy the position of the aorta and, as a result, will arise from the left ventricle posteriorly.*

Morphologically, the heart in uncomplicated transposition differs in two respects from the normal heart: not only do the two great arteries arise from the 'wrong' ventricles, but their antero-posterior relationship is reversed as well. *We therefore have the interesting situation in which the term 'transposition' can be taken to mean that the great arteries are transposed, as far as their ventricular origin is concerned, or that they are transposed relative to each other.* This is undoubtedly one major reason why over the years so many attempts have been made to formulate a satisfactory definition that not only would be applicable for the uncomplicated malformation, but also would retain its validity in the presence of associated anomalies. In 1963 I defined transposition of the great arteries (3) as 'that condition in which the aorta lies anterior to the pulmonary trunk and originates from a morphologic right ventricle anterior to the crista supraventricularis or its remnant,' and added that 'the pulmonary artery (trunk) may originate from either ventricle or override a defect'. I believe that this definition is still a valid one. It might be refined somewhat by replacing the term 'its remnant' by 'its equivalent'.

There are two reasons why the origin of the pulmonary trunk is not really important for the diagnosis of TGA, e.g., in cases associated with a ventricular septal defect (VSD): 1) the embryological error which causes reversal in position of the great arteries takes place distal to the conus cordis (vide infra), and 2) from a developmental point of view both arteries are right sided, i.e., they initially arise from the primitive right ventricle. The arterial interrelationship in tetralogy of Fallot and double outlet right ventricle (DORV) is essentially normal, and nobody at present would consider these two anomalies forms of TGA, even though the aorta originates wholly or in part from the right ventricle. By the same token, the posteriorly positioned pulmonary trunk may originate from the right ventricle in cases of transposition, either completely (and separated from the mitral valve by a band of muscle in which case we are dealing with a combination of two defects: TGA and DORV), or partially (with pulmonary-mitral fibrous continuity) representing a combination of TGA and tetralogy of Fallot. Also, whether or not a ventricular septum is present is, in my opinion, not important, and I believe it to be unwise to change the name of an anomaly just because another cardiac anomaly is present. Not even the form of DORV in which there is an anteriorly located subpulmonary VSD with the pulmonary trunk (in levoposition) overriding the defect (Taussig-Bing heart), is considered a form of TGA, even though the aorta originates wholly from the right ventricle and the pulmonary trunk in part from the left ventricle (4-7). There is little or no functional difference between this lesion and TGA with a posterior VSD and overriding pulmonary trunk. It is not surprising, therefore, and rather unfortunate, that that anomaly at one time was also referred to as Taussig-Bing anomaly – erroneously, as Beuren (5) and others have pointed out.

I believe that the lesion in which the aorta arises from the right ventricle (right posteriorly) and the pulmonary trunk from the left ventricle (left anteriorly – the so-called 'posterior transposition'), pathogenetically is related to DORV, and has nothing to do with the classical form of TGA. It simply represents the end-stage of the series: DORV with posterior VSD (usual type of DORV) → DORV with anterior VSD and levoposition of the pulmonary trunk (Taussig-Bing heart) → heart with an aorta arising from the right ventricle posterior and to the right of a pulmonary trunk which originates from the left ventricle in an anterior position ('posterior transposition'). The explanation for this is as follows: if the levoposition of the pulmonary trunk goes far enough, then there comes a point at which the embryonic conal septum comes to lie in the same plane as the muscular ventricular septum and fuses with it, either completely, with, as a result, an intact ventricular septum, or in part, in which case a ventricular septal defect of varying size remains. It makes no difference to the embryo with what the conal septum fuses. It, the conal septum, consists of endocardial cushion tissue and if it comes into contact with other endocardial cushion tissue (e.g., that present along the upper border of the muscular ventricular septum) it can fuse with it.

Similarly, if, in the above series, TGA is associated (in the sense that the two arteries are transposed relative to each other), then we have the series: DORV with posterior VSD and TGA → DORV with anterior VSD, TGA and levo-position of the aorta → DORV with pulmonary trunk arising from the right ventricle in a posterior position, and the aorta originating from the left ventricle in an anterior position (so-called 'anatomically corrected TGA'). It is important to realize that in both 'posterior TGA' and in 'anatomically corrected TGA' it is the *anterior* portion of the embryonic conus cordis which becomes transferred to the left ventricle, not the posterior half as in the normal.

As in all forms of DORV, the muscle separating the tricuspid valve from the right posterior great artery is the infundibulo-ventricular fold (the equivalent of the embryonic cono-ventricular fold), not the crista supraventricularis. There is no crista supraventricularis in these hearts since the infundibular septum, which is normally incorporated into the crista supraventricularis, has been 'used' to complete the ventricular septum. It is furthermore to be expected, as in all forms of DORV, that both the arterial valves are separated from the mitral valve by muscle (infundibulo-ventricular fold).

What, then, is the pathological anatomy of classical transposition of the great arteries? In the uncomplicated form (for the purposes of this discussion I will limit myself to uncomplicated TGA), as stated above, the aorta arises anteriorly from the right ventricle, anterior and somewhat to the right of the crista supraventricularis. The pulmonary trunk arises from the left ventricle posterior and usually slightly to the right or the left of the ascending aorta, while its valve occupies the position of the aortic valve in the normal heart. The leftward position of the pulmonary trunk may, at times, be quite pronounced, in which case the aortic arch courses over the right pulmonary artery rather than the left. The aortic valve is somewhat further to the right than is the pulmonary valve of the normal heart and faces to the right and superior, rather than to the left superior and posterior. The atria and the ventricles are anatomically perfectly normal. This suggests to me that the embryological error which leads to TGA takes place distal to the conus cordis. I should like to emphasize at this point that a transposition heart should *not* be compared anatomically with the normal heart of an older infant or child but with the heart of a newborn. The reason for this is obvious: since the right ventricle in TGA has to sustain systemic pressures it will retain the right ventricular hypertrophy present in the newborn. In other words, the differences that we see in the transposition heart are the result of different hemodynamics and, therefore, of a secondary nature. The same is true for the abnormal position of the aortic valve in transposition to which I referred above.

This also is a secondary, hemodynamically-induced abnormality, since the right ventricle empties into the ascending aorta, the long axis of which is similar to that of the normal heart, i.e., directed to the right and superior, whereas the long axis of the pulmonary trunk in the normal is directed to the left, superior and posterior. In congenital aortic atresia the pulmonary trunk and ductus arteriosus assume a course similar to that of the ascending aorta and aortic arch in transposition (8). In these cases the pulmonary valve occupies a position virtually identical to that of the aortic valve in transposition of the great arteries.

In looking at hearts with uncomplicated transposition of the great arteries in newborns I have always been struck by the fact that these specimens look so 'normal' and neat. There is no thickening of valves, nor are there any other features which would immediately suggest abnormality.

Although we do not know what the pathogenesis of transposition is, certain observations can be made which give us a clue as to what may have happened in a general sense: 1) The majority of cases of transposition of the great arteries are uncomplicated and in an additional, significant percentage of cases, there is only a minor associated anomaly; 2) inversion of the ventricles, or so-called L-loop (corrected TGA) heart, is almost always associated with transposition of the great arteries.

These two observations suggest to me that the basic development error in transposition of the great arteries not only is a simple, single one, but also that it represents an either/or situation (6). In other words: the embryo has the choice between using one of two developmental processes; either the normal one which results in a normal heart, or the abnormal one which results in transposition. Since the ventricles anatomically are normal I believe the developmental abnormality to take place somewhere distal to the conal septum. The embryo either uses the intercalated valve cushions to partition the truncus arteriosus (these cushions becoming the major ones, while the normal truncus cushions remain small and simply form a valve cusp each), or the aorticopulmonary septum develops on the left instead of the (normal) right side. Each of these two pathogenetic mechanisms would result in transposition of the great arteries. It is even conceivable that one or the other mechanism may have been operative in a particular case of TGA. As has been alluded to above, there are cases of TGA in which the pulmonary trunk is located posterior or posterior and slightly to the right of the aorta with the aortic arch coursing over the left pulmonary artery, and others in which the pulmonary trunk is located rather far to the left and only slightly posterior to the aorta with the aortic arch crossing the right pulmonary artery. The first variant could be explained on the basis of an inverted development of aortico-pulmonary septum, the second one could be due to the intercalated valve cushions becoming the major cushions dividing the truncus arteriosus rather than the truncus cushions which remain small and simply form a valve cusp.

The first mechanism could explain why, in cases of L-loop, the arteries are usually transposed. The aorticopulmonary septum in these cases develops normally since it lies extrapericardially, while the ventricles, the conal septum and the truncal septum all develop in mirror image of normal. Therefore the result, of necessity, will be a transposed position of the arteries. In order for the two great arteries to be normally interrelated and to arise from their proper ventricle (in an anatomic sense) in cases of L-loop, a second anomaly is necessary, i.e., that anomaly, whatever it may be, which in the D-loop results in transposition of the great arteries (7).

All of this, obviously, is rather speculative and undoubtedly will remain so until such time that we are in a position to study the pathogenesis of TGA in embryologic material, as has been done recently with respect to other cardiovascular anomalies (9, 10).

REFERENCES

1. Van Praagh, R., Perez-Trevino, C., Lopez-Cuellar, M. et al., Transposition of the great arteries with posterior aorta, anterior pulmonary artery, subpulmonary conus and fibrous continuity between aortic and atrioventricular valves. *Am. J. Cardiol.* 28, 621 (1971).
2. Farre, J. R., On malformations of the human heart. In: *Pathological Researches*, Essay 1, London 1814.
3. Van Mierop, L. H. S., Wiglesworth, F. W., Pathogenesis of transposition complexes. II. Anomalies due to faulty transfer of the posterior great artery. *Am. J. Cardiol.* 12, 226 (1963).
4. De la Cruz, M. C., Da Rocha, J. P., An ontogenetic theory for the explanation of congenital malformations involving the truncus and conus. *Am. Heart J.* 51, 282 (1956).
5. Beuren, A., Differential diagnosis of the Taussig-Bing heart from complete transposition of the great vessels with a posteriorly overriding pulmonary artery. *Circulation* 21, 1071 (1960).
6. Van Mierop, L. H. S., Wiglesworth, F. W., Pathogenesis of transposition complexes. III. True transposition of the great vessels. *Am. J. Cardiol.* 12, 233 (1963).
7. Van Praagh, R., What is the Taussig-Bing malformation? *Circulation* 38, 445 (1968).
8. Van Mierop, L. H. S. and Gessner, I. H., Pathogenetic mechanisms in congenital cardiovascular malformations. *Prog. Cardiovasc. Dis.* XV(1), 67 (1972).
9. Van der Linde-Sipman, J. S., *Het links hypoplastisch hart bij de minipig*, Thesis Utrecht 1977.
10. Van Mierop, L. H. S., Patterson, D. F. and Schnarr, W. R., Hereditary defects of the conotruncal septum in Keeshond dogs: Embryologic studies. *Am. J. Cardiol.* 40, 936 (1977).

13. CONSIDERATIONS PERTINENT TO THE EMBRYOGENESIS OF TRANSPOSITION

A. C. G. WENINK

Obviously, full explanation of the problem of transposition must still be awaited. To the discussion presented in the preceding chapters, the present author will add only a few additional considerations. These will largely be based upon two different observations.

The first observation to be reported is concerned with the notion that transposition of the great arteries is a malformation of the outflow portion of the heart. During embryonic development, much of the internal architecture of the arterial end of the heart consists of endocardial swellings. These are the truncal ridges and, below the future arterial orifices, the bulbar ridges. Fusion of the left and right bulbar ridges gives rise to the bulbar septum. The proximal portion of the right bulbar ridge is anterior to the future tricuspid orifice, and it not only contributes to the crista supraventricularis but also to the anterior leaflet of the tricuspid valve. The proximal part of the left bulbar ridge partly continues along the trabecula septomarginalis and partly lies on the rim of the ventricular septum, to continue posteriorly in the tissue of the atrioventricular sulcus (1). These tissues are of a very plastic nature and can easily be subject to secondary influences. It has been observed, that haemodynamics can greatly influence the development of these endocardial swellings (2). Thus, any comparison between the normal architecture of the embryonic heart and the morphology of fully developed malformed hearts cannot be made with certainty. It is not known in what way certain influences might have transformed the endocardial masses during development of congenital malformations. Nevertheless, discussions on congenital cardiac malformations have centred round these endocardial masses. The abnormal position of the infundibular septum in a series of malformations has been amply commented upon by Anderson et al. (3). Inversion of the left and right bulbar ridges in transposition has been assumed by Lev and Saphir (4). Goor and Edwards (5) actually thought that they could observe such an inversion in pathological specimens.

In literature, descriptions of malformed embryonic hearts are extremely rare. Therefore, some words may be devoted to a double outlet right ventricle in a human embryo of 16 mm crown-rump length, of which a full description is in preparation. In this embryo, both arteries arise from the future right ventricle, and in addition an endocardial mass is present between the outflow region of the left ventricle and the right sided aorta, indicating the improbability of a mere delay of transfer of the aorta to the left ventricle. The endocardial ridge under discussion cannot be diagnosed as either the left or the right bulbar ridge. Rather it seems to be an abnormal connection between the two bulbar ridges. Form and site of the bulbar septum are not in keeping with the developmental stage. Any growth of the abnormal ridge could perhaps have completed the bulbar septum, but would at the same time have sealed off the aortic outlet. In the present context, this observation is mentioned to illustrate the relative difficulty in correlating normal embryonic, with abnormal fully developed structures. When this difficulty exists concerning endocardial cushion tissue, it is felt to be less disappointing to consider the ventricular septum, which is a muscular structure right from its earliest appearance. Too many cases of transposition of the great arteries show abnormalities of the ventricular septum, for the opinion to be upheld that the form and site of the septum is not related to the pathogenesis of transposition. The data presented here concern 150 cases of transposition of the great arteries, defined as ventriculo-arterial discordance without other abnormal connections. Half of the cases possessed in addition one or more ventricular septal defects (see Oppenheimer-Dekker, this book, page 139). The anomaly of the ventricular septum mentioned consists of an abnormal position. In addition, its anterior portion was often thicker than in the normal heart. From the right side, the infundibulum was seen to be less deep than normal, and it would appear that the anterior septum portion had not its normal leftward curve. However, seen from the left, this curve was almost always present. Some cases even showed leftward deviation of the septum; that is, an exaggerated leftward curve. Some cases suffered from pulmonary stenosis as a result of this septal displacement, as described by Van Gils elsewhere in this book. The abnormal position of the septum was still better illustrated by its posterior portion. The septum could be said to have rotated rather than shifted, for its posterior portion was in many cases deviated to the right. This rightward deviation brought a separate component of the septum into view. This component, called the posteromedial muscle, remained at its usual site on the posterior ventricular wall, its base originating just between the atrioventricular orifices, while the rest of the septum had a less constant position. The posteromedial muscle was not always equally well distinguishable. Its presence was noted in 35% of the cases with an intact ventricular septum. A frequency of 80% was noted in the cases of transposition with ventricular septum defect. In 56 normal hearts, only twice a posteromedial muscle was seen.

It is thought that the posteromedial muscle is a direct consequence of septation of the atrioventricular canal. Principally, it has nothing to do with ventricular septation proper. Invagination of the posterior part of the atrioventricular canal has a congruent influence on the directly related portions of the heart, i.e. the posterior walls of atrium and ventricle (fig. 1). This means,

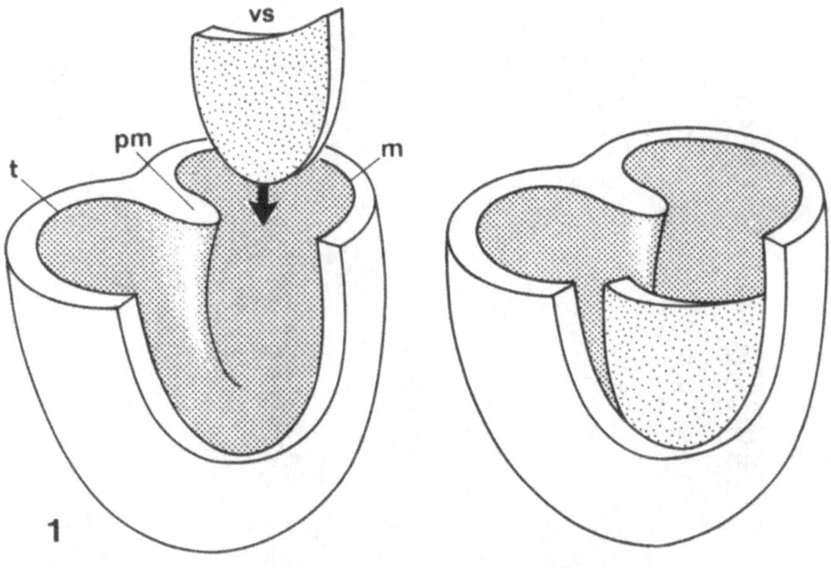

Figure 1. Diagram to show the rightward deviation of the ventricular septum (vs) which is independent of the postero-medial muscle (pm). The latter maintains a constant position relative to the mitral (m) and tricuspid (t) orifice.

that proper septation of the atrioventricular canal in the absence of ventricular septation would leave a muscular ridge on the posterior ventricular wall. Indeed, such a ridge has been noted in cases of 'single ventricle' and 'common ventricle' (6). It was described as a portion of the true posterior ventricular septum and as a posterior median ridge respectively. Similarly, such a ridge has been observed in hearts with transposition and a straddling tricuspid valve, in which it was called a dorsomedian muscle ridge (7). Actually, these

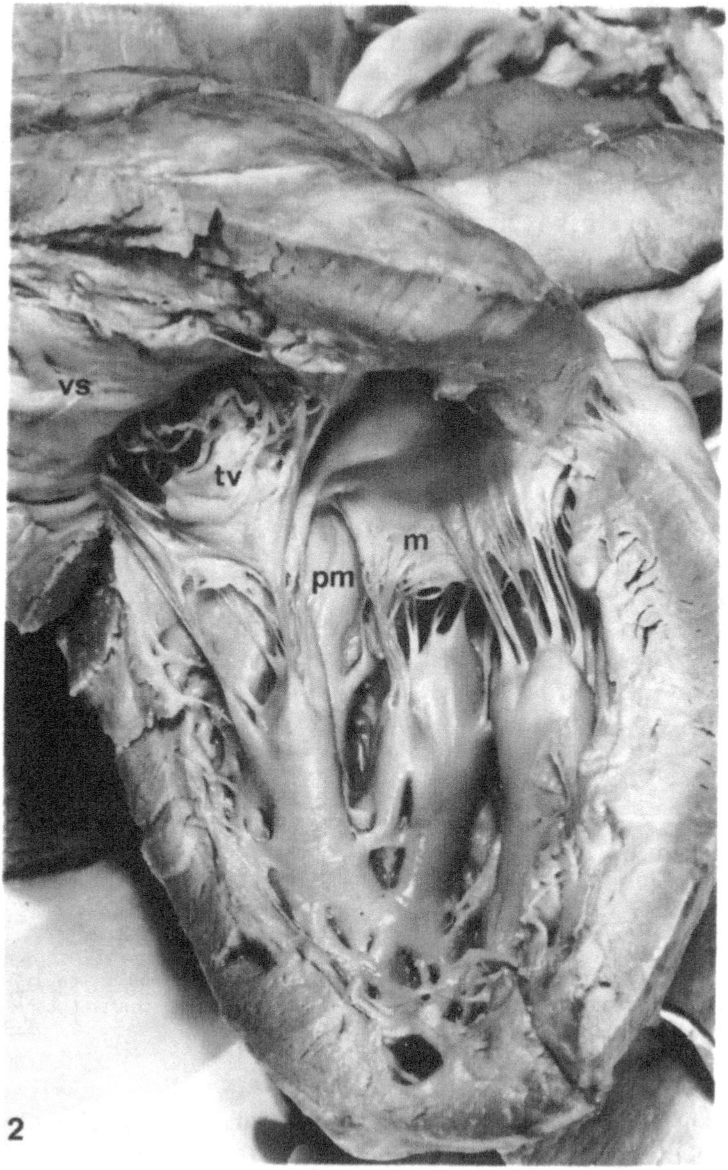

Figure 2. Left ventricular view of a case of transposition with straddling of the tricuspid valve (tv). The posteromedial muscle (pm) is between the tricuspid and mitral (m) valves and has no relation with the ventricular septum (vs).

latter cases are an extreme example of rightward deviation of the posterior part of the septum. Here, the posteromedial muscle can be easily distinguished, because it is widely separated from the rest of the septum, and part of the tricuspid valve is between the two (fig. 2). In less extreme cases, the poste-

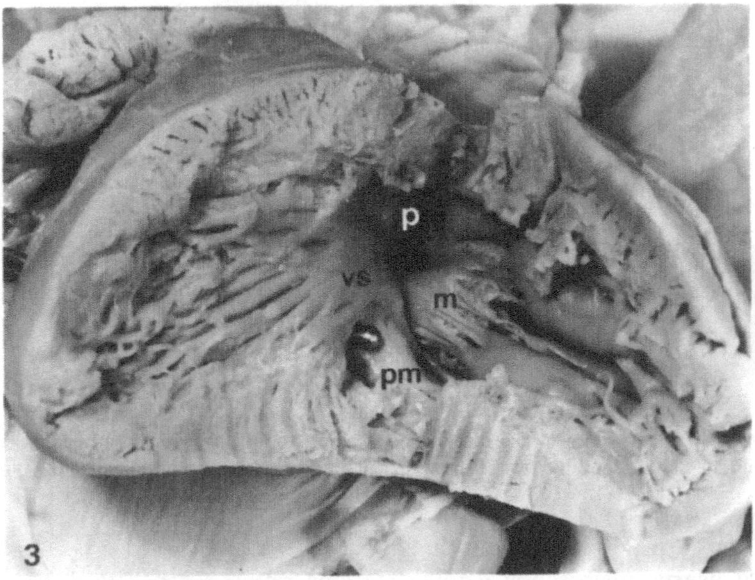

Figure 3. Left ventricular view of a case of transposition. A probe is visible in the ventricular septal defect between the posteromedial muscle (pm) and the rest of the ventricular septum (vs). m: mitral valve; p: pulmonary orifice.

romedial muscle is separated from the rest of the septum by a conspicuous, often slitlike ventricular septal defect (fig. 3). From the right, tricuspid valvular tissue can be seen to adhere to the rim of the defect. Sometimes, only a groove is present between the posteromedial muscle and the ventricular septum. In these cases it would seem as if the posteromedial muscle is an unusual trabeculation, which is apposed to the left side of the septum (fig. 4).

As a consequence of the above observations, it is suggested that transposition of the great arteries is not merely an outflow malformation. At any rate, a great number of cases show a lack of correspondence of the septational processes in the ventricle and the atrioventricular canal.

Possibly, this correspondence is always subject to slight variations. For in

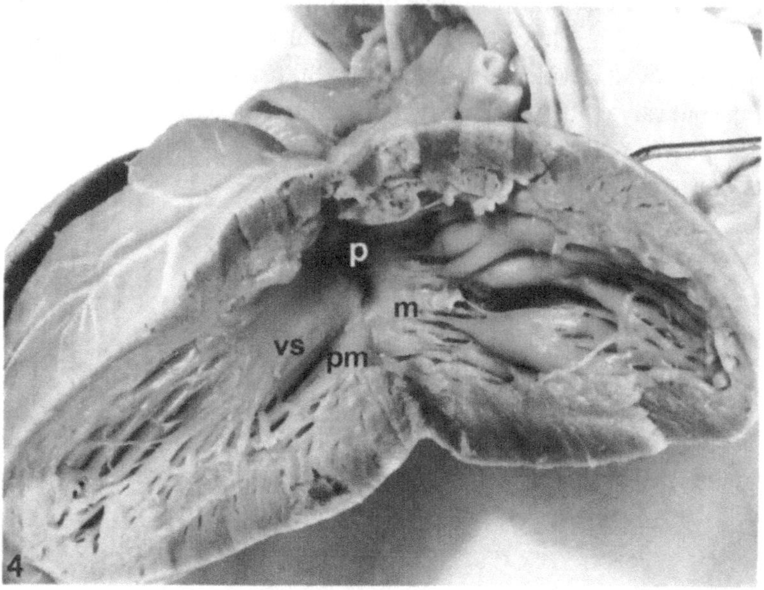

Figure 4. Left ventricular view of a case of transposition, to show the groove between the posteromedial muscle (pm) and the rest of the ventricular septum (vs). m: mitral valve; p: pulmonary orifice.

foetal hearts, microscopical investigations reveal a separate dorsal component of the ventricular septum (see Gittenberger-De Groot and Wenink, this book, pag. 15). A possible hypothesis is that this separate structure is loosened from the septum in those anomalies in which the septum turns away from its normal site relative to the atrioventricular canal.

In conclusion, transposition of the great arteries is considered to be the result of a comprehensive developmental process. Developmental correlations between the atrioventricular region and the arterial pole of the heart are of paramount importance. Such correlations have been previously denoted by Shaner (8) and Doerr (9).

REFERENCES

1. Wenink, A. C. G., *Some details on the final stages of heart septation in the human embryo.* Thesis Leiden 1971.
2. Pexieder, T., Cell death in the morphogenesis and teratogenesis of the heart. *Advances Anat., Embryol. and Cell Biol.* 51-3 (1975).

3. Anderson, R. H., Wilkinson, J. L., Arnold, R., Becker, A. E. and Lubkiewicz, K., Morphogenesis of bulboventricular malformations II. Observations on malformed hearts. *Br. Heart J.* 36, 948 (1974).
4. Lev, M. and Saphir, O., Transposition of the large vessels. *J. Techn. Methods* 17, 126 (1937).
5. Goor, D. A. and Edwards, J. E., The spectrum of transposition of the great arteries, with special reference to developmental anatomy of the conus. *Circulation* 68, 406 (1973).
6. Lev, M., Liberthson, R. R., Kirkpatrick, J. R., Eckner, F. A. O. and Arcilla, R. A., Single (primitive) ventricle. *Circulation* 39, 577 (1969).
7. Devloo, A. and Ritter, D. G., A dorsomedian muscle ridge between both atrioventricular valves in transposition of the great vessels. *7th Europ. Congr. Cardiology*, Abstr. Book II, 56 (1976).
8. Shaner, R. F., Malformation of the atrioventricular endocardial cushions of the embryo pig and its relation to defects of the conus and truncus arteriosus. *Am. J. Anat.* 84, 431 (1949).
9. Doerr, W., Über ein formales Prinzip der Koppelung von Entwicklungsstörungen der venösen und arteriellen Kammerostien. *Z. Kreislaufforsch.* 41, 269 (1952).

PART II

TRANSPOSITION OF THE GREAT ARTERIES

B. Morphological aspects

14. INTERVENTRICULAR COMMUNICATIONS IN TRANSPOSITION OF THE GREAT ARTERIES

A. OPPENHEIMER-DEKKER

INTRODUCTION

It has become apparent for quite some time that the formulation of a clear definition for the congenital cardiovascular anomaly, generally known as transposition of the great arteries, proves to be more difficult than its simple name would suggest. This holds even more true for transposition with interventricular communications (a term used here in preference to 'ventricular septal defects', for reasons, which will be explained in the part 'Anatomical description'). Actually (as is also indicated by Van Mierop, this book, page 123) one can easily be led astray by this very terminology, since the word 'transposition', taken in its literal sense, emphasizes the interrelationship of the great arteries, while in practice it is usually and rather loosely considered to be interchangeable with the condition in which the aorta arises from the right ventricle and the pulmonary trunk from the left ventricle. As Beuren (1, 2) rightly pointed out, previous classifications of transposition of the great arteries were based either on anatomical or clinical grounds. It is obvious, that intermingling or inaccurate handling of the concepts readily causes confusion.

In the past the usual inclination was to identify the anomaly with (and reduce it to) the one characteristic of the abnormal arterial interrelationship, the ascending aorta arising from the heart anterior to the pulmonary trunk, with these vessels pursuing a course parallel to each other. This feature is indeed conspicuous on external inspection of a specimen or, clinically, on the angiocardiograms. And of course it is true that in pure, uncomplicated forms, consistent with the commonly accepted clinical notion of transposition, this arterial interrelationship is one of the decisive characteristics. However, even this feature appeared to raise controversies.

Until about 10 years ago, misunderstandings and misinterpretations remained limited, basically confined to debates among experts about the essentials of the anomaly, scattered relatively scarcely in the scientific journals, and thus not affecting the whole world of cardiology. Most people agreed that the reversal in position should not be taken so literally as to imply a 180-degree change in the location of the orifices (which Grant (3) proved to be wrong by roentgenographic measurements). Confusion, however, grew and increased accordingly as during the last decade or so lengthy and detailed discussions of the question which malformation really deserved the name 'transposition of the great arteries', became regular ingredients in the table of contents of the scientific journals. A climax in the 'stir-up' was reached, when Van Praagh et al. (4) introduced the transposition with posterior aorta and anterior pulmonary artery, and several of his colleagues tried to clear the air (5, 6), during which period the term 'posterior transposition' was born. Interestingly enough more than 8 years before Van Praagh's c.s. provocative publication Mehrizi and Taussig (7) reported two cases of what they called complete transposition of the great vessels, in which at autopsy '. . . the great vessels occupied their normal position . . .' (case 1) or '. . . the pulmonary artery occupied its normal position, that is, anterior and to the left of the aorta and the aorta lay to the right and slightly more anterior than its normal position . . .' (case 2). In both cases their anatomical diagnosis was transposition of the great vessels (with ventricular septal defect), because '. . . it was found that the aorta arose from the right ventricle and the pulmonary artery was seen to arise mainly from the left ventricle . . .'. The authors did not really give attention to the fact, that the great vessels occupied their normal position nor did it occur to them to call this malformation 'posterior transposition'. Yet it seems worthwhile to quote this paper, on the one hand because it is an instructive example of loosely intermingled clinical and anatomical reasoning, on the other hand because, apparently, these authors back in 1963 unintentionally described two cases of this currently so disputed anomaly.

GENERAL COMMENTS

If now, with these introductory remarks in mind, we concentrate upon the subject interventricular communications in transposition, we have to consider the context of this book with the foregoing chapter devoted to various ways of looking at the pathogenesis of transposition connected with differing views on terminology. Therefore, although not wittingly avoiding any reference to embryology, we do not select an approach stressing the embryopathogenetic significance (as was recently done by Thiene et al. (8)). The main goal is to set forth several anatomical features, which are considered important for obtaining insight into the intraventricular morphology in cases of transposition with interventricular communication. In this respect one logical question is of course the incidence of this combination. There is considerable variation in the percentages given by the various authors, which seems to depend not only on the definition chosen by the investigators, but probably even more on the period of time during which the post mortem material was collected. When the present author reported on transposition in 1962 (9), a period in which the possibilities for surgical procedures were very limited, and consequently infants with uncomplicated transposition had hardly any chance to survive, her group of 45 specimens comprised 30 cases without other anomalies (except for patency of the foramen ovale or the ductus arteriosus) and 15 cases with interventricular communication. This is in keeping with other publications of those years (10, 11, 12). The figures of Edwards (13) in 1969, mentioning the presence of a ventricular septal defect in about one third of the cases, seem to be influenced by his definition of transposition, referring to any developmental abnormality in the relationship between the positions of the aorta and pulmonary trunk (for this very reason he included his display on transposition in a chapter named 'Malformations of the thoracic aorta'). With the onset of modern heart-surgery, the percentage of uncomplicated transpositions in post mortem collections decreased proportionately, but there can be little doubt that the over-all incidence of uncomplicated transposition amply exceeds that of transposition with interventricular communications.

In our investigation we did not include the cases with complex associated anomalies like atresia of a cardiac orifice, atrioventricular discordance, univentricular hearts. However, our cases with interventricular communications dò cover specimens with overriding pulmonic ostium, provided that the degree of overriding appeared to be definitely less than 50%. These criteria are the same as those of 1962 (9) and resulted now in a material of 75 cases, among a total collection of 150 specimens with, in the terminology of Anderson (this book, page 93), 'ventriculo-arterial discordance and atrioventricular concordance'.

ANATOMICAL OBSERVATIONS

In the first columns of table 1 the position of the ascending aorta as related to the pulmonary trunk is schematically represented, both for the group with and for the group without interventricular communication (for the entire material of 150 transposition hearts the percentages can thus be calculated as follows: at the right and anterior in 66%, at the right side by side 19%, anterior in 10%, at the right and posterior in 5%). It should be noted, that in our specimens with the aorta situated at the right and posterior to the pulmonary trunk, the location of the aorta was always slightly more anterior than its normal position. Furthermore, we appreciate, that some of our cases, registered in the subgroup 'aorta anterior to the pulmonary trunk', would be classified by several other investigators (14) as 'complete levotransposition of the great arteries'. We also realize, that some cases with the great vessels side by side would by some authors (15) be labeled as 'partial distortion of the great vessels'. However, for the reasons, mentioned above, the purely descriptive basis for presenting the various features will obtain priority in this contribution.

As to the location of the defects, the descriptive startingpoint requires a combined definition of the right and left ventricular characteristics with regard to this location. This approach undoubtedly hampers a streamlined, unequivocal categorization, but benefits, however, the recognition of the interdependence of right and left ventricular as well as septal morphology. It also allows for marking off several main lines as presented in the following survey, which for practical purposes places the right ventricular view, before the left ventricular view.

For the description of the interventricular communications a division in three main groups is made. Group I, covering the right ventricular outflow tract, is quantitatively the largest group and includes various types. Group II comprises the atrioventricular level and group III is related to the muscular part of the ventricular septum below the outflow tract.

Group I. The majority of the interventricular communications is found to have a relation with the infundibular part of the ventricular septum. In normal hearts this can be roughly indicated as the crista supraventricularis with the septal band (16), but recently the terms 'infundibular septum' and 'trabecula septomarginalis' have been proposed for an infundibular nomenclature, applicable to both normal and malformed hearts (17). Adopting this terminology, the representatives of this group can be defined as the result of either an incomplete development of these structures or an incomplete junction between them and the rest of the septum. For obvious reasons, the incomplete junction will be, in a number of cases, the consequence of an incomplete development in the sense of deficiency in substance, but this is not the general rule.

Within the limits of the forementioned broad definition, both the nature

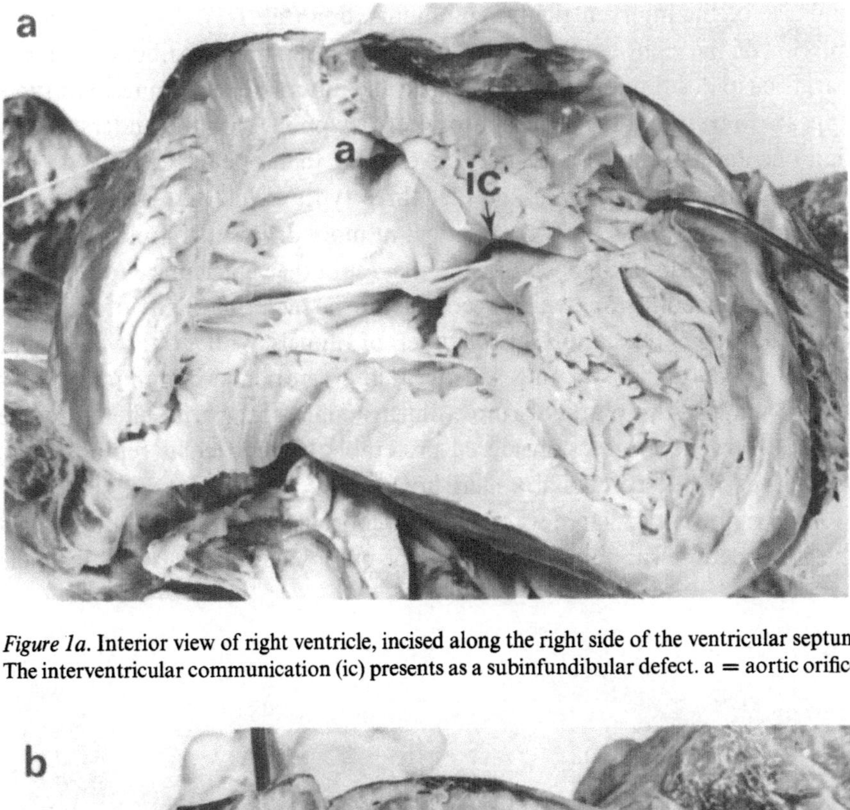

Figure 1a. Interior view of right ventricle, incised along the right side of the ventricular septum. The interventricular communication (ic) presents as a subinfundibular defect. a = aortic orifice.

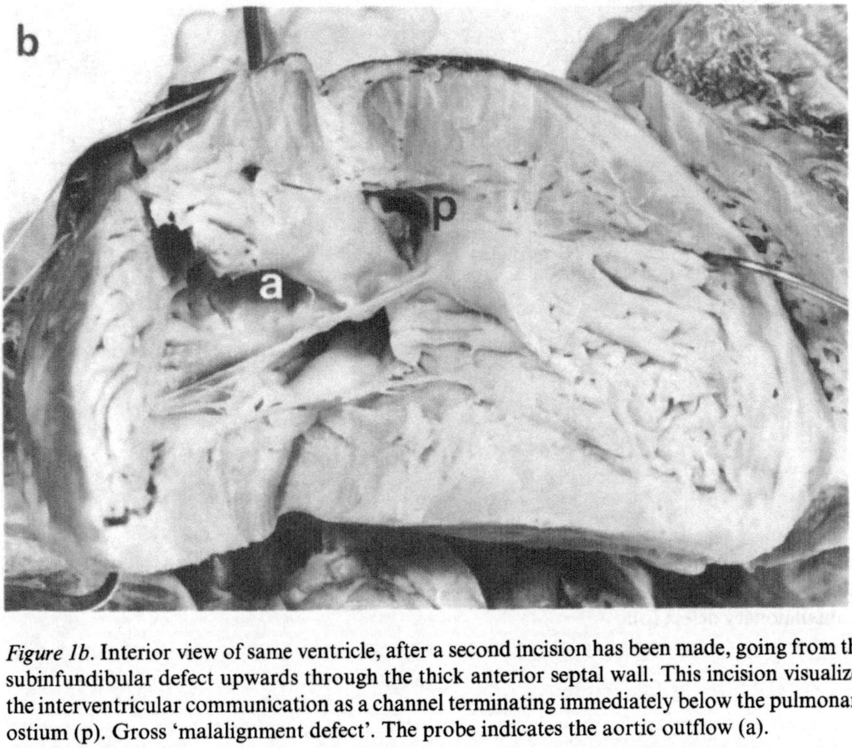

Figure 1b. Interior view of same ventricle, after a second incision has been made, going from the subinfundibular defect upwards through the thick anterior septal wall. This incision visualizes the interventricular communication as a channel terminating immediately below the pulmonary ostium (p). Gross 'malalignment defect'. The probe indicates the aortic outflow (a).

and the degree of incompleteness provide a large-scale variety in localization and size of the interventricular communication (fig. 1-5). As seen from the interior of the right ventricle, a categorization in subinfundibular, anterior paratricuspid, subpulmonary, subaortic and antero-superior muscular types appears to be useful from the anatomical viewpoint, with the understanding that one and the same defect may cover more than one of these types. This overlap affects in particular the first three types (which are also the most commonly encountered) as the product of more or less incomplete junction between the infundibular septum and the rest of the ventricular septum. This is also the phenomenon, which accounts for the fact, that many of the interventricular communications are channels or tunnels, with a right ventricular and a left ventricular opening. The term interventricular communication is used to indicate this markedly three-dimensional appearance. Therefore, the term is for general use, considered preferable to ventricular septal defect, which is easily interpreted as a mere hole.

If the right ventricular view of an interventricular communication permits the qualification 'subpulmonary', then the pulmonary orifice is usually over-

C

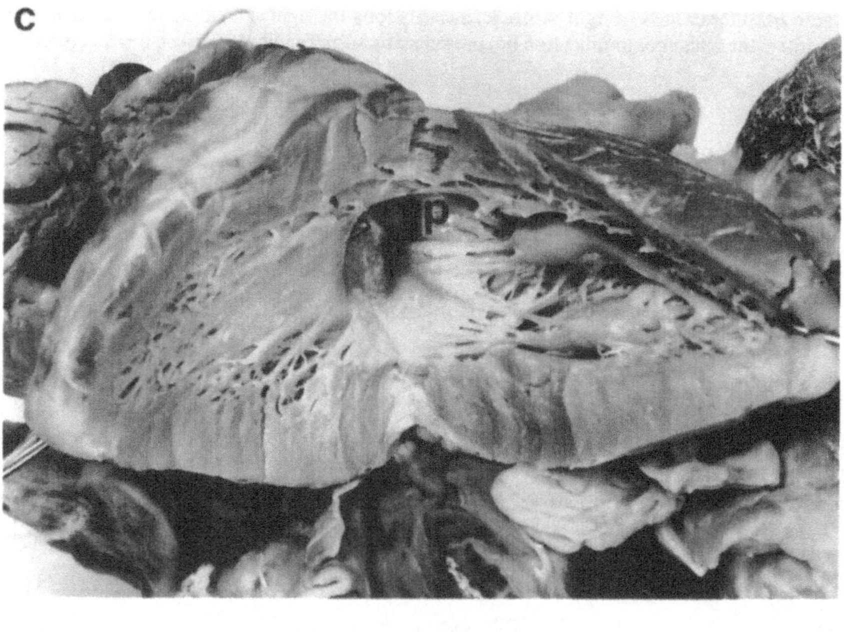

Figure 1c. Same specimen, interior view of left ventricle, incision made along the left side of the ventricular septum. The interventricular communication, indicated by a probe, presents as a subpulmonary defect (p).

riding. Occasionally it may be a combined subaortic-subpulmonary type, with adjacent aortic and pulmonary semilunar cusps, but with the pulmonary orifice arising completely from the left ventricle. A leftsided subpulmonary defect corresponds with different localizations on the right ventricular side; quite often this is subinfundibular or paratricuspid (fig. 1 and 2).

a

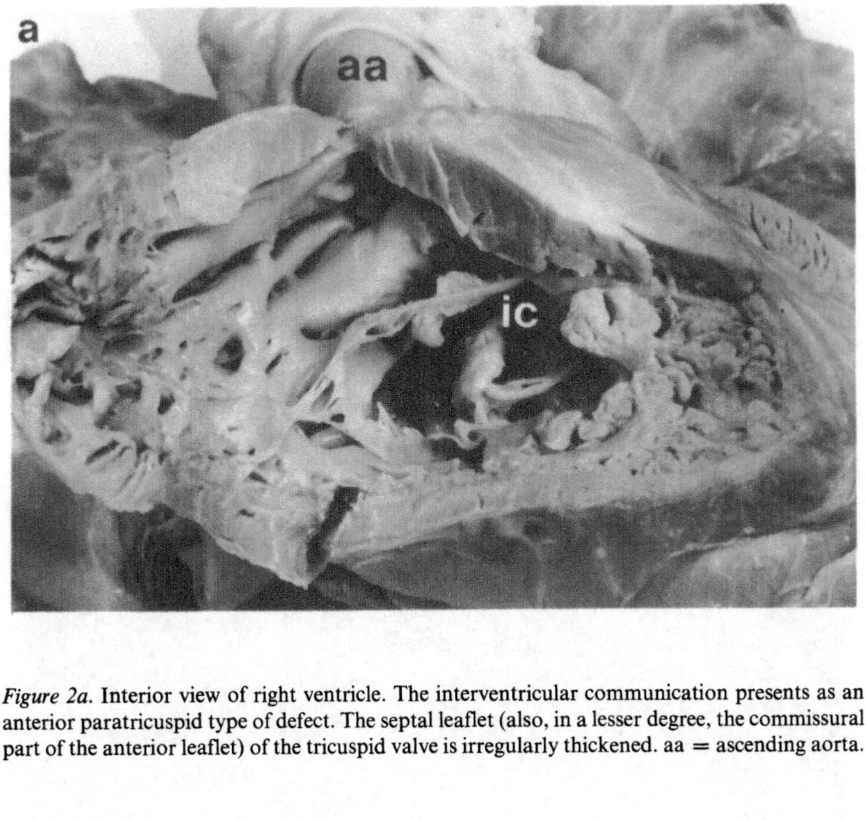

Figure 2a. Interior view of right ventricle. The interventricular communication presents as an anterior paratricuspid type of defect. The septal leaflet (also, in a lesser degree, the commissural part of the anterior leaflet) of the tricuspid valve is irregularly thickened. aa = ascending aorta.

The subaortic type appears to be rather variable in its left ventricular presentation, which is, among other things, related to where the defect borders on the aortic orifice, and over what distance this occurs. If it is in the neighbourhood of the anterior and left semilunar cusps, both right and left ventricular views will show a high localization (fig. 3). However, if it is adjacent to the right and/or posterior cusps, the left ventricular position will tend to the paramitral (fig. 4 and 5). As is shown in the pictures, this may result in conspicuous differences in left ventricular morphology. Not infrequently a

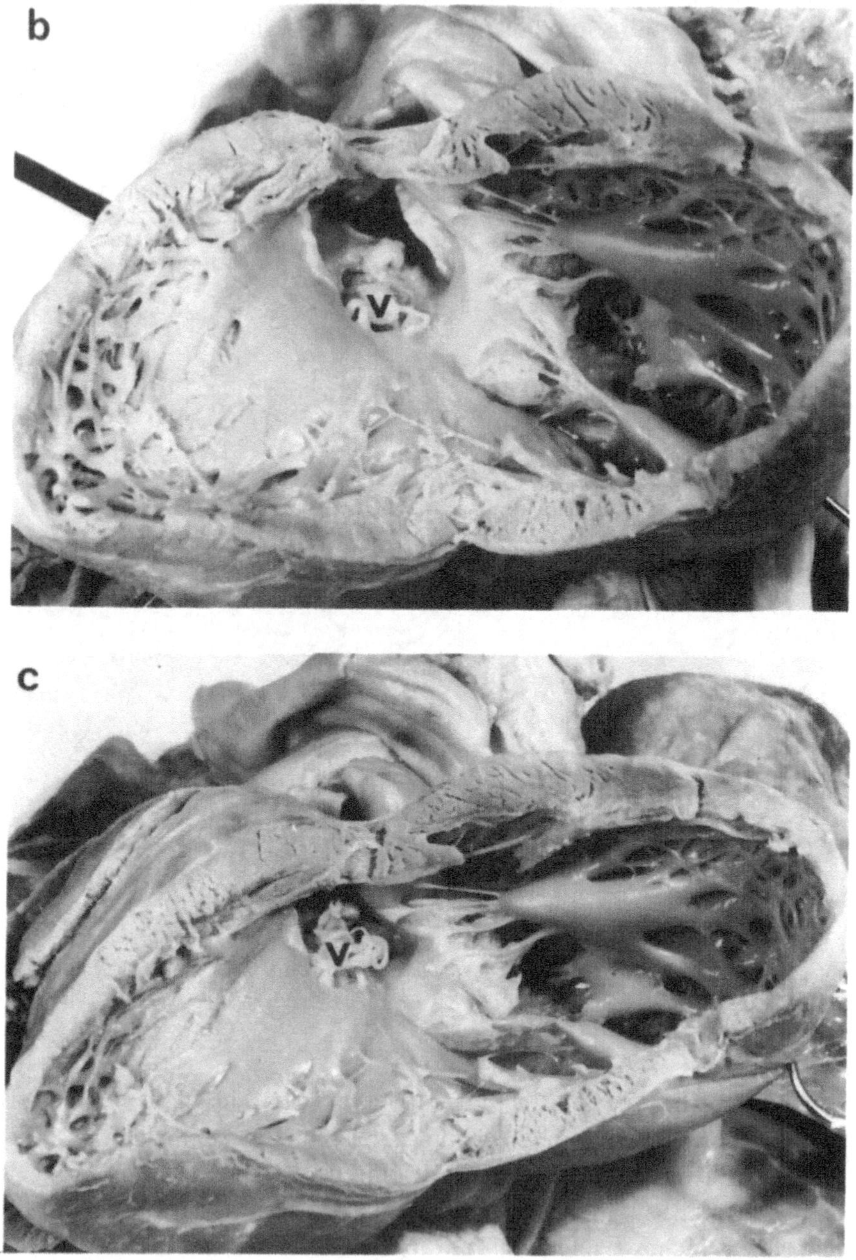

Figure 2b and c. Same specimen, interior views of left ventricle. The subpulmonary defect is filled with a protruding mass of redundant tricuspid valvular tissue (v).

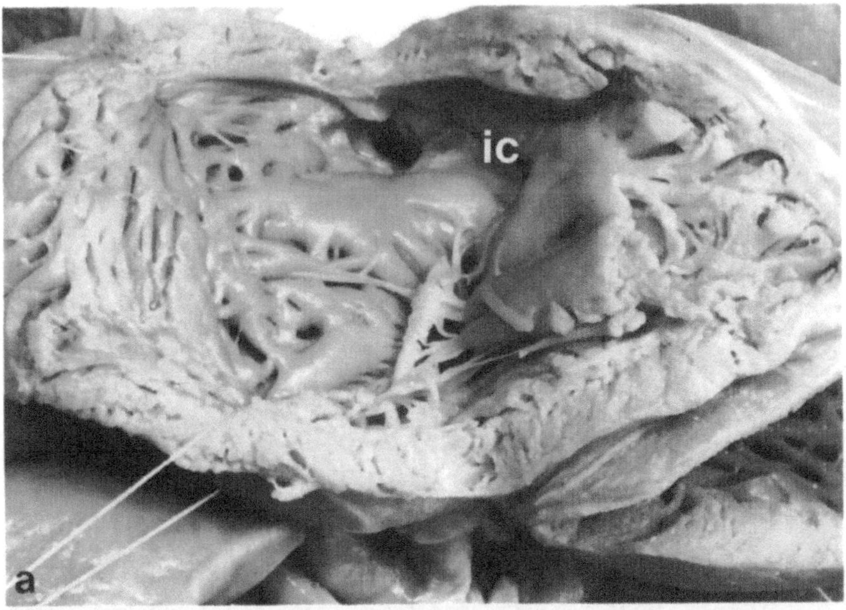

Figure 3a. Interior view of right ventricle. The anterosuperior part of the subaortic interventricular communication is adjacent to the left aortic semilunar cusps. Its posterior border is formed by a pronounced muscle bundle, crossing the ventricular septum, thus extending in the left ventricular cavity.

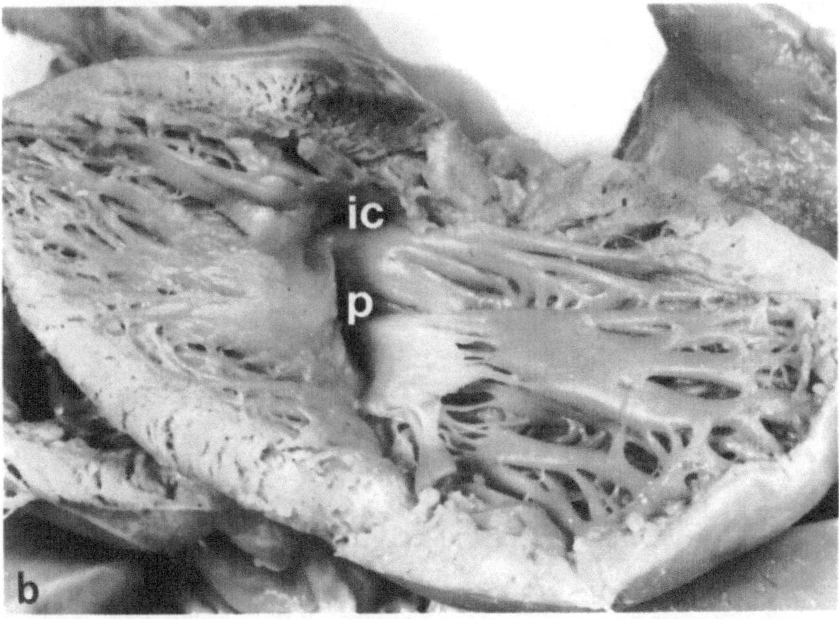

Figure 3b. Same specimen, interior view of left ventricle, showing a high level of the interventricular communication. Its posterior border, indicated in fig. 3a, extends anterior to the pulmonary ostium, which consequently has a relatively posterior position (in this case combined with a narrowing of its entrance, see van Gils, this book, page 160).

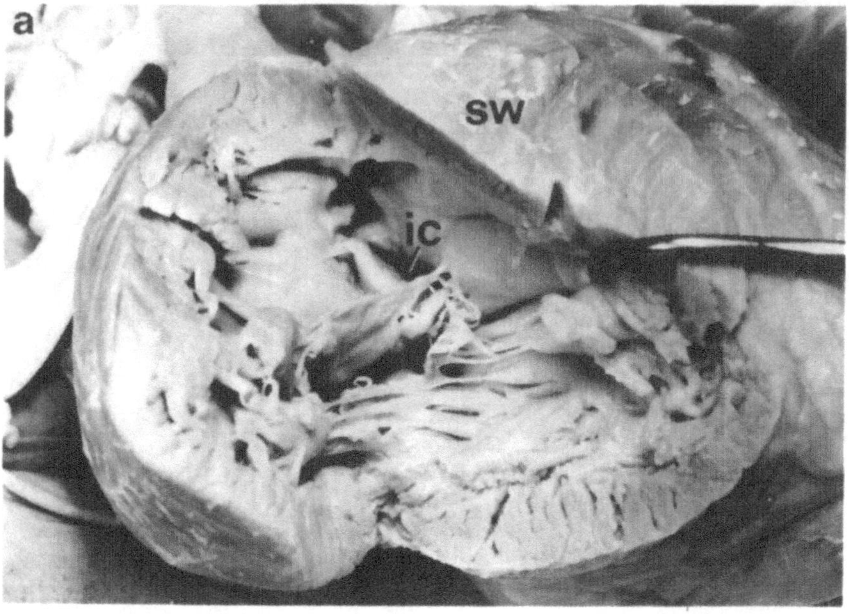

Figure 4a. Interior view of right ventricle. The subaortic interventricular communication borders on the posterior aortic semilunar cusp. Note the broad anterior septal wall (sw).

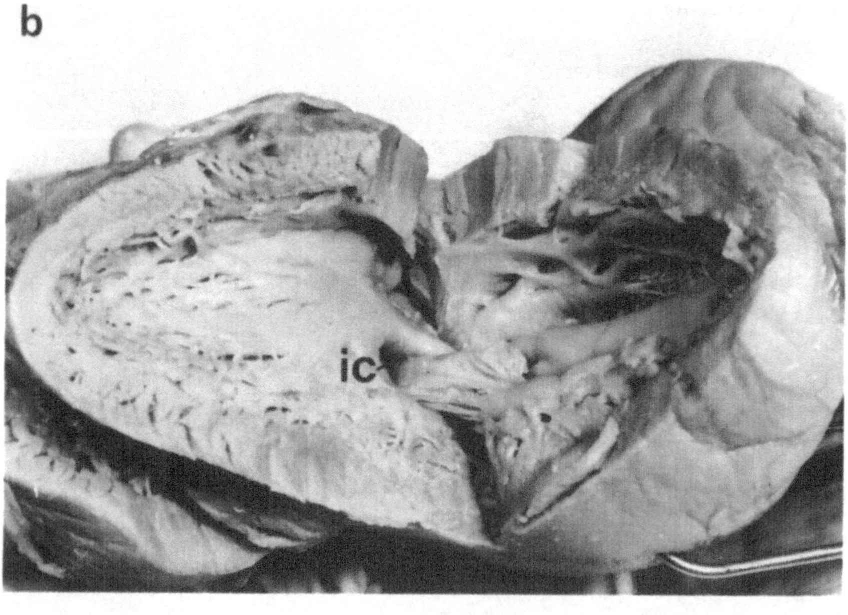

Figure 4b. Same specimen, interior view of left ventricle. Paramitral position of the interventricular communication, pulmonary orifice easily accessible.

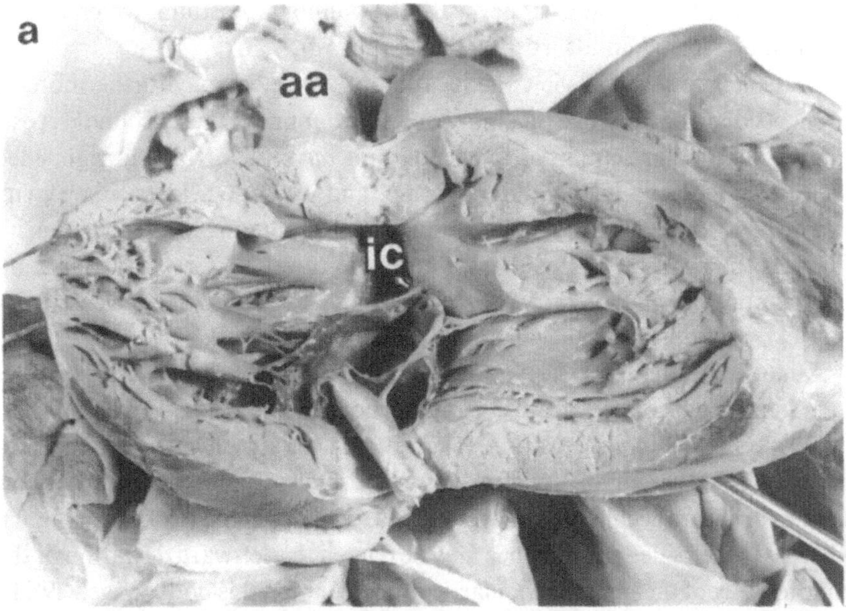

Figure 5a. Anterior view of right ventricle. The subaortic interventricular communication, posterosuperiorly bordering on the right and posterior aortic semilunar cusps, represents a gap between parietal and septal walls of the infundibulum. The tip of a probe, situated in the lower part of the left ventricular cavity, is visible immediately anterior to the tricuspid valve.

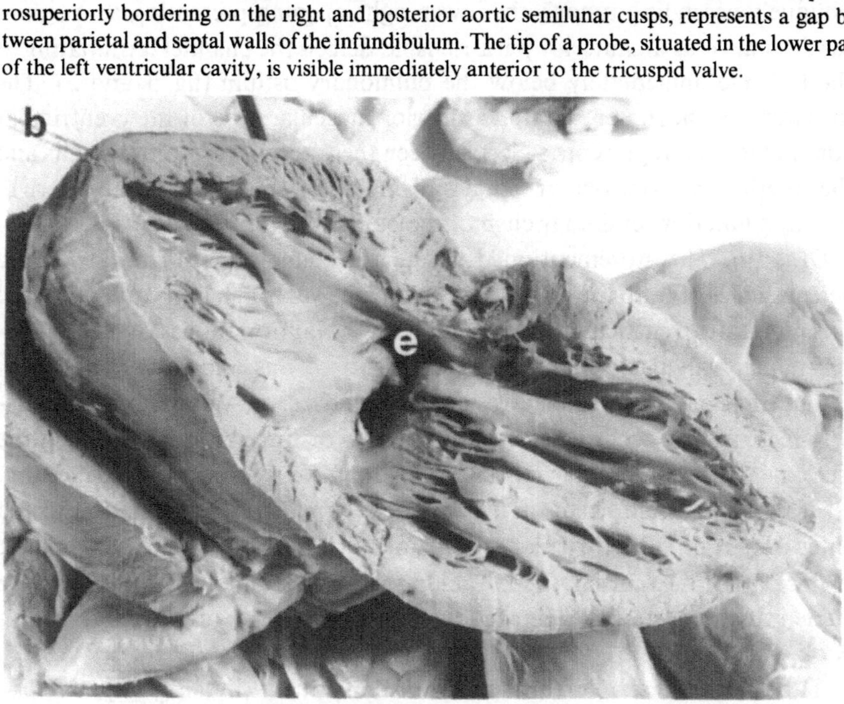

Figure 5b. Same specimen, interior view of left ventricle. Paramitral localisation of the interventricular communication (indicated by the tip of a probe). Note the septal excavation (e) below the pulmonary orifice.

septal excavation is found underneath the pulmonary ostium, which at first sight can be mistaken for a septal defect (fig. 5b).

In the left ventricular view the location of the defect may furthermore be influenced by the presence of a more or less pronounced muscle bundle crossing the ventricular septum as a boundary of the septal defect, in rightsided continuity with the infundibular septum, and in the left ventricular cavity extending either anteriorly or posteriorly to the pulmonary ostium. This influences the position of this ostium in relation to the interventricular communication and the mitral valve (fig. 3b) and can cause a left ventricular outflow tract obstruction (van Gils, this book, page 160).

A marked difference in level between the right and left openings of the interventricular communication can also be brought about by another feature, a sometimes considerably thickened anterior septal wall. This thickening may be either right- or leftsided; in the first instance the infundibular septum or the trabecula septomarginalis participates in the thickening (fig. 1), whereas the leftsided prominence may be related to a leftward deviation of the anterior part of the interventricular septum (Wenink, this book, page 129). In such a broad thickening an interventricular communication can extend as an obliquely ascending tunnel, the lower right opening presenting as a subinfundibular or as an anterior paratricuspid defect, the channel terminating at the left side immediately below the pulmonary ostium (fig. 1 and 2). The infrequently encountered antero-superior muscular type of interventricular communication represents a cleft between the trabecula septomarginalis and the anterior right ventricular septal wall; in the left ventricle it is found close to the right anterior semilunar cusp of the pulmonary orifice.

Group II. The aforementioned, frequently found, anterior paratricuspid defect shades off into the group, resembling the ventricular type of the partial common atrioventricular canal anomaly. Malformations of the atrioventricular valvular apparatus forming part of this anomaly, include coherent tricuspid and mitral valves, overriding tricuspid valve (sometimes hardly recognizable, characterized only by two or three chordae crossing the free edge of the ventricular septum) or cleft anterior mitral valve leaflet (fig. 6). If this latter malformation is combined with a leftward deviation of the anterior part of the ventricular septum and an adherence of the mitral leaflet to this part of the septum, then the entrance to the pulmonary orifice may be hidden at the postero-inferior side of the cleft mitral valve (van Gils, this book, page 160).

In this respect it should be emphasized, that not only in this group, but also in the other forms of transposition with interventricular communication, the mitral region is conspicuously variable (fig. 6 and 7).

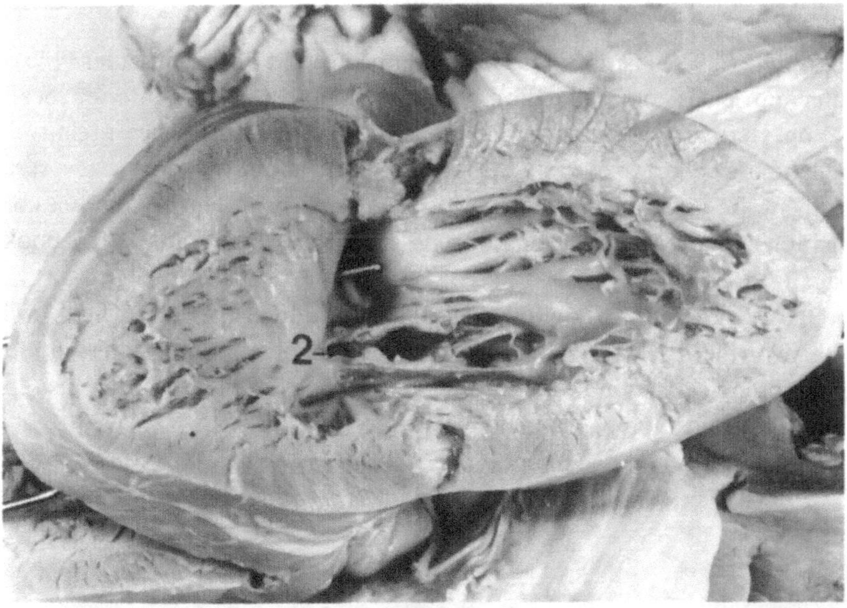

Figure 6. Interior view of left ventricle. A subpulmonary interventricular communication is indicated by a probe. A second communication (2), resembling the ventricular type of the partial common atrioventricular canal anomaly is hidden between the cleft parts of the anterior mitral valve leaflet, attached to the interventricular septum.

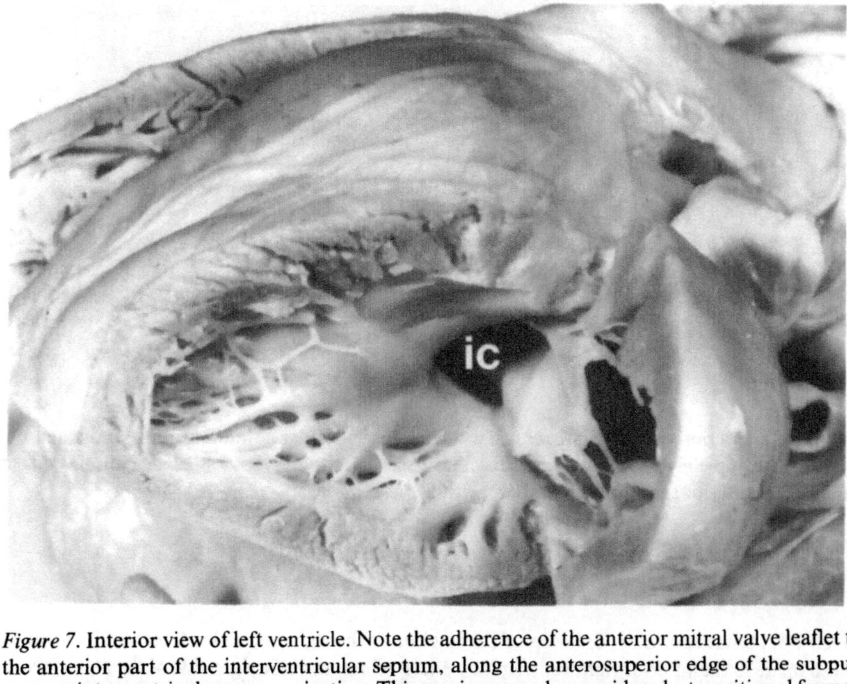

Figure 7. Interior view of left ventricle. Note the adherence of the anterior mitral valve leaflet to the anterior part of the interventricular septum, along the anterosuperior edge of the subpulmonary interventricular communication. This specimen can be considered a transitional form to the cases, in which the pulmonary orifice is hidden at the postero-inferior side of the cleft mitral valve.

Group III. The last group to be mentioned is that of the muscular type of interventricular communication with a central or a postero-inferior localization. Here I shall confine myself to remarking that the incidence is relatively high (in our collection we found 13 examples, i.e. about 17%) and that several of them are associated with a defect of group I or group II. The possible relationship with the embryopathogenesis is discussed by Wenink (this book, page 129).

One of the specimens, with a central localization of the defect (fig. 8) will receive further attention in the part 'The membranous septum', in the scope of a microscopical investigation into the morphology of the membranous septum in transposition of the great arteries.

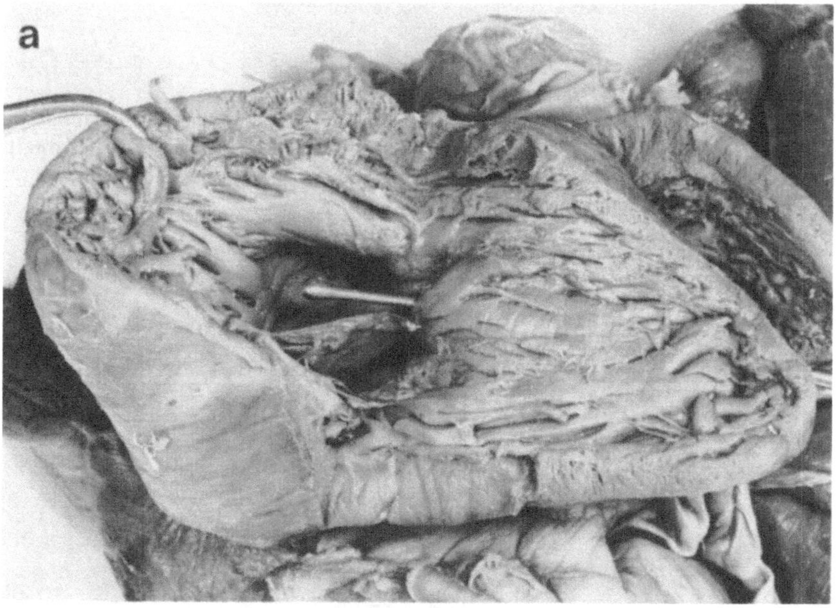

Figure 8a. Interior view of right ventricle. The interventricular communication, indicated by a probe, is completely surrounded by muscular tissue. The right ventricular incision has cut the thickened anterior septal wall (compare with fig. 8c).

Figure 8c. Same specimen, drawing of the interior of the right ventricle. A second incision has been made in the anterior right ventricular wall, terminating at the right side of the aortic orifice.

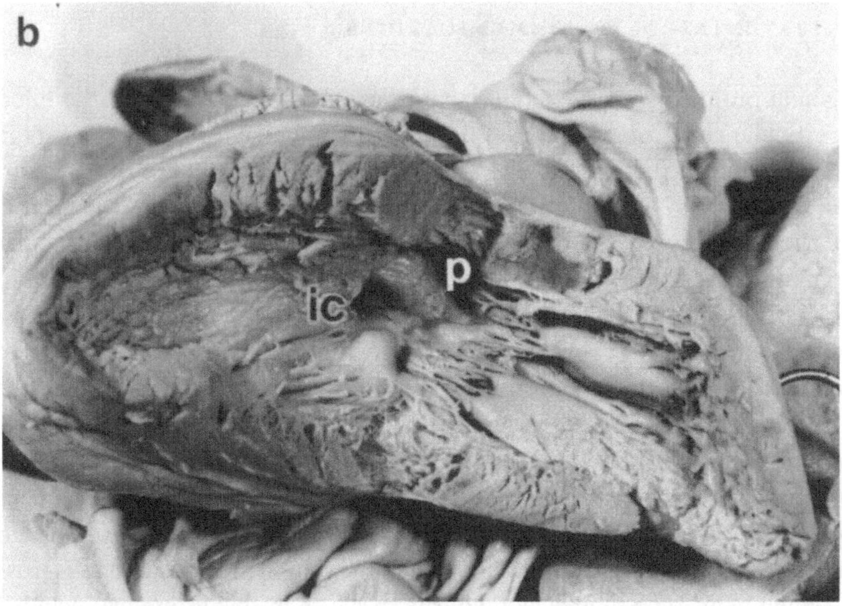

Figure 8b. Same specimen, interior view of left ventricle. The interventricular communication is separated from the pulmonary and mitral valves by muscular tissue.

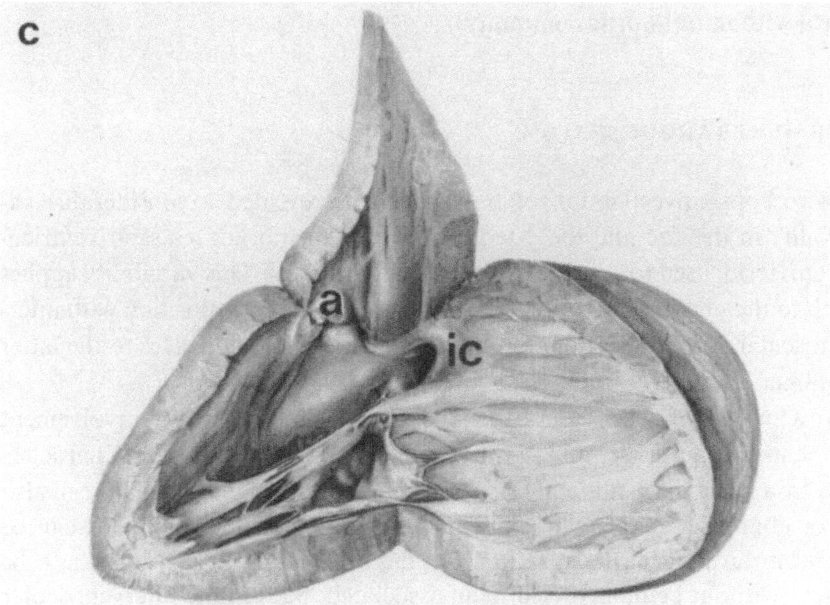

ARTERIAL INTERRELATIONSHIPS AND LOCALIZATION OF INTERVENTRICULAR COMMUNICATIONS

Having outlined some main characteristics of the topography of the interventricular communications the question arises whether or not there exists an interdependence between their localization and the position of the great arteries. Although we could not find a *strict* correlation between the arterial interrelationship on the one hand and the location of the interventricular communication on the other, it was possible to attach a certain amount of predictive value to the position of the great arteries, as is shown in the last columns of table 1. It is worth mentioning, that in the group with the most common type of arterial interrelation (aorta to the right and in front of the pulmonary trunk) a majority had the paratricuspid type of interventricular communication, and that in the relatively small group with anterior aorta the subaortic type was frequently found (in our material we had 12 specimens with the subaortic type, and 5 of these cases belonged in the group with anterior aorta!). It is not surprising, that in the side-to-side position the 'gross malalignment' type figures as favourite, because in this group we included cases with (mild to moderate) overriding of the pulmonary ostium. The small group with slightly posterior aorta showed no preferential type (although the assumed 'posterior' transposition (6) is described as having an overriding aorta with mitral-aortic continuity).

THE MEMBRANOUS SEPTUM

Macroscopic investigation of our specimens revealed a considerable variability in the size and the extent of the pars membranacea septi ventriculorum (term, used for the first time by Reinhard (18)). This variability applies both to the uncomplicated transposition and to the transposition with interventricular communication, but here we shall confine ourselves to the latter combination.

In a number of cases, described in the groups I and II there was involvement of the membranous septum in the septal defect. Other cases were characterized by a more than moderate size of the membranous septum. This can also be of abnormal shape, can show aneurysma-like proliferations, or can be found in an unusual localization. On the other hand, it can appear to be absent without being involved in an associated, but remote interventricular communication. In particular this latter observation must be considered insufficiently proven by macroscopic study alone. Therefore, several transposition hearts were serially sectioned, and microscopically compared with identically serially sectioned, normal foetal and neonatal hearts.

This study produced conclusive evidence of the occasional absence of the membranous septum (which is also, rather casually, mentioned by Bharati and Lev (19) in a study on the conduction system in hearts with transposition). The pars membranacea septi in the literal sense should be found in continuity with the right fibrous trigone and with the right wall of (in transposition hearts) the pulmonary trunk in such a way that the lowest semilunar cusp should be attached to this thin membrane. In figure 9a-e transverse sections are shown of a specimen with a central muscular type of interventricular communication (cf. fig. 8). These sections demonstrate, that the annulus fibrosus near the pulmonary ostium has an irregular contour, that the lower posterior part of the ostium, i.e. the lower semilunar cusp, is indeed continuous with the annulus fibrosus, but that the membranous septum to be expected as a thin fibrous structure between the left ventricle and right atrium (atrioventricular part) and between the left and right ventricles (interventricular part) is missing. In its place a thick muscle mass can be recognized

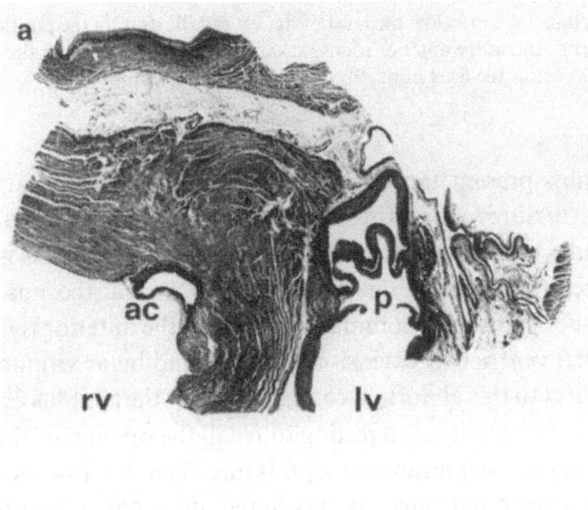

Figure 9a. Transverse section at the level of the pulmonary orifice and the left posterior aortic semilunar cusp (ac). lv = left ventricle, rv = right ventricle.

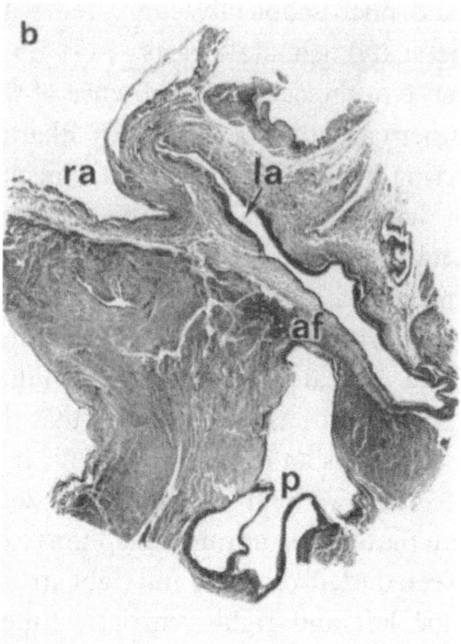

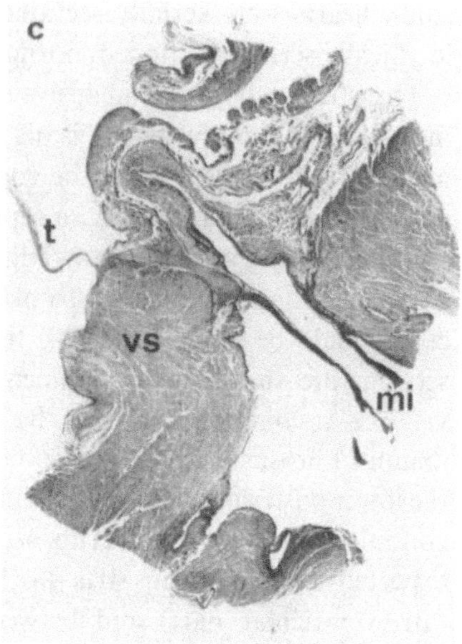

Figure 9b. Section, 3,5 mm below the level of fig. 9a, immediately underneath the posterior pulmonary semilunar cusp, through the adjacent part of the annulus fibrosus (af). The wall separating the left ventricle from the right atrium (ra) and from the right ventricle is thick and muscular. la = left atrium.

Figure 9c. Section 2.8 mm below the level of fig. 9b and illustrating the position of both mitral valve leaflets (mi) and of the anterior tricuspid valve leaflet (t), which were already present in the section 0.9 mm below the level of fig. 9b. No membranous septum.

which remains present throughout the sections until it separates into two muscular structures bordering the interventricular communication: the muscle bundle between the tricuspid and mitral valve leaflets is the posteromedial muscle (see Wenink, this book, page 129), while the muscle bundle between the interventricular communication and the anterior right ventricular wall is the left ventricular extension of the infundibular septum.

With respect to this abnormal configuration of the annulus fibrosus and the membranous septum it is interesting to recall the opinion of Bochdalek (20), that the term pars membranacea septi is mistaken, because, according to his view, the structure indicated by this name, does not belong to the septum cordis, but should be considered as the root of the aorta (in normal hearts), as it is developmentally a part of the left and the right annulus fibrosus.

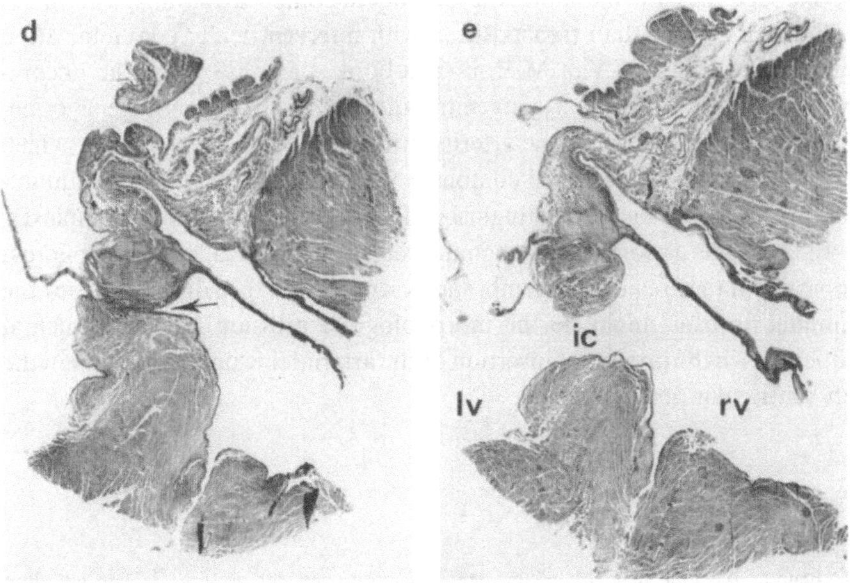

Figure 9d. Section 0.7 mm below the level of fig. 9c, through the upper border of the interventricular communication (arrow).
Figure 9e. Section at the level of the interventricular communication.

In connection with the aforementioned proliferations found in the region of the membranous septum, clear-cut aneurysms appeared to be rare in our material and our microscopical studies indicated that it is usually redundant tissue of the septal tricuspid leaflet which protrudes beneath the pulmonary ostium (cf. fig. 2).

CONCLUDING REMARKS

Although transposition with interventricular communication appears, morphologically, frequently characterized by definitely abnormal outflow tracts, it should be realized, that this abnormal architecture itself need not, of necessity, represent the primary pathogenetic factors in the development of 'ventriculo-arterial discordance'. Certain features of left ventricular septal and atrioventricular valve morphology, as outlined above, point to the hypothesis, that anomalous development in the inflow region might play a part in the pathogenesis of this and other malformations (Wenink, this book, page 129). Furthermore, the fact that uncomplicated transposition has a higher incidence than transposition with interventricular communication supports the view of Van Mierop (this book, page 123), that the uncomplicated transposition is a congenital anomaly with the pathogenetic mechanism situated distal to the arterial orifices and that this anomaly (which can of course secondarily be combined with an interventricular communication) should be sharply distinguished from other transposition complexes.

Finally, the abnormalities encountered macroscopically and/or microscopically in the area of the membranous septum and the adjacent part of the annulus fibrosus might be the morphologic expression of developmental difficulties in the process of insertion of the arterial (i.e. pulmonic) root in the left ventricular outflow tract.

REFERENCES

1. Beuren, A., Eine neue Einteilung der Transpositionen der grossen Gefässe und ihre Differentialdiagnose. In: *Proceedings of the third European Congress of Cardiology*, Rome, 1960.
2. Beuren, A., Differential diagnosis of the Taussig-Bing heart from complete transposition of the great vessels with a posteriorly overriding pulmonary artery. *Circulation* 21, 1071 (1960).
3. Grant, R. P., The morphogenesis of transposition of the great vessels. *Circulation* 26, 819 (1962).
4. Van Praagh, R., Pérez-Trevino, C., López-Cuellar, M., Baker, F. W., Zuberbuhler, J. R., Quero, M., Pérez, V. M., Moreno F. & Van Praagh, S., Transposition of the great arteries with posterior aorta, anterior pulmonary artery, subpulmonary conus and fibrous continuity between aortic and atrioventricular valves. *Am. J. Cardiol.* 28, 621 (1971).
5. Van Mierop, L. H. S., Transposition of the great arteries. Clarification or further confusion? *Am. J. Cardiol.* 28, 735 (1971).
6. Wilkinson, J. L., Arnold, R., Anderson, R. H. & Acerete, F., 'Posterior' transposition reconsidered. *Br. Heart J.* 37, 757 (1975).
7. Mehrizi, A. & Taussig, H. B., Acyanotic transposition of the great vessels. *Bull. Johns Hopkins Hosp.* 112, 239 (1963).
8. Thiene, G., Razzolini, R. & Dalla-Volta, S., Aorto-pulmonary relationship, arterioventricular alignment and ventricular septal defects in complete transposition of the great arteries. *Eur. J. Cardiol.* 4, 13 (1976).
9. Dekker, A., Transposition of the great vessels. In: *Proceedings of the fourth World Congress of Cardiology*, Mexico, 1962.
10. Elliott, L. P., Neufeld, H. N., Anderson, R. C., Adams, P. & Edwards, J. E., Complete transposition of the great vessels I. An anatomic study of sixty cases. *Circulation* 27, 1105 (1963).
11. Sherman, F. E., *An atlas of congenital heart disease*. Philadelphia 1963.
12. Edwards, J. E., Carey, L. S., Neufeld, H. N. & Lester, R. C., *Congenital heart disease.* Philadelphia/London 1965.
13. Edwards, J. E., Congenital malformations of the heart and great vessels, H. Malformations of the thoracic aorta. In: Gould, S. E. (ed.), *Pathology of the heart and blood vessels.* Springfield Illinois 1968.

14. Lincoln, C., Hasse, J., Anderson, R. H. & Shinebourne, E., Surgical correction in complete levotransposition of the great arteries with an unusual subaortic ventricular septal defect. *Am. J. Cardiol.* 38, 344 (1976).
15. Angelini, P. & Leachman, R. D., Pulmonary artery originating anteriorly from the left ventricle. *Am. J. Cardiol.* 32, 840 (1973).
16. Van Mierop, L. H. S., Anatomy and embryology of the right ventricle. In: Edwards, J. E., Lev, M. & Abell, M. R. (ed.), *The Heart*, Baltimore 1974.
17. Anderson, R. H., Becker, A. E. & Van Mierop, L. H. S., What should we call the 'crista'? *Br. Heart J.* 39, 856 (1977).
18. Reinhard, H., Zur anatomischen und pathologischen Kenntnis der dünnen Stelle in der Herzscheidewand (Pars membranacea septi ventriculorum). *Virchows Arch. pathol. Anat. u. Physiol.* 12, 129 (1857).
19. Bharati, S. & Lev, M., The conduction system in single, regular (d-), complete transposition with ventricular septal defect. *J. Thorac. Cardiovasc. Surg.* 72, 194 (1976).
20. Bochdalek, jr., Anatomische Beiträge. Zur Anatomie des menschlichen Herzens. I. Über die sogenannte pars membranacea septi ventriculorum cordis. *Arch. Anat. Physiol. wiss. Med.*, 320 (1868).

Table 1. Interrelationship ascending aorta-pulmonary trunk in 150 specimens with transposition

	75 without I.C.	75 with I.C.	Preferential type I.C.
1) 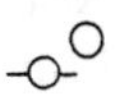	60 (80%)	39 (52%)	paratricuspid
2) 	5 (6%)	24 (32%)	gross malalignment
3) 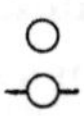	8 (11%)	7 (10%)	subaortic
4) 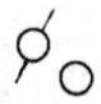	2 (3%)	5 (6%)	no preferential type

Explanation of the symbols:
I.C. : Interventricular Communication
1) : aorta at the right and anterior to pulmonary trunk
2) : aorta and pulmonary trunk side by side
3) : aorta anterior to pulmonary trunk
4) : aorta at the right and slightly posterior to pulmonary trunk

15. LEFT VENTRICULAR OUTFLOW TRACT OBSTRUCTION IN TRANSPOSITION WITH INTERVENTRICULAR COMMUNICATION: ANATOMICAL ASPECTS

F. A. W. VAN GILS

In the normally developed human heart the outflow tract of the left ventricle is wide and easily accessible. Certain structures, as infundibular septum and anterolateral muscle bundle of the left ventricle, if present, do not obstruct this outflow tract, nor do any of the surrounding valvular structures. However, in malformed hearts, like those with transposition, it is not uncommon that such structures cause an obstruction, either alone or in combination with other factors. The obstruction can result in a pulmonary stenosis at subvalvular or valvular level. This paper will be restricted to obstructions at the subvalvular level, which often occur in cases of transposition with ventricular septal defect. This is indicated in the literature for if cases with other complex intracardiac malformations are excluded, the incidence of left ventricular outflow tract obstruction ranges from 7 to 25 percent of transposition cases autopsied, with an average of 16 percent (1-9). It goes without saying that an obstruction may vary from a simple one to a combination of several abnormal structures and situations as there are muscular structures in malalignment and septal bulging, membranous structures – either redundant mitral or tricuspid valvular tissue or proliferations of the membranous septum – and abnormal attachments and connections (1-3, 6-19).

Recently, the author and colleagues (2) published their observation, that malalignment septal defect occurred in about half of their cases with transposition and interventricular communication. Subvalvular pulmonary stenosis was shown in more than half of the specimens in this latter group. Thus, it is not surprising to find from an overall review of the literature that one third of cases with transposition, interventricular communication and subvalvular pulmonary stenosis appeared to show a malalignment defect. A problem in this respect is the interpretation of the descriptions, which often make it difficult to determine the exact nature of the outflow tract obstruction and sometimes even the existence or the type of an interventricular communication. Moreover, many descriptions were given before the term 'malalignment' was introduced.

Bulging of the ventricular septum is also frequently described; the pulmonary stenosis resulting from this type of muscular obstruction is less severe than in cases with a muscular obstruction brought about in malalignment.

Subvalvular fibromuscular stenosis has often been described either as a diffuse 'tunnel' type or as a localized 'ring' or 'diaphragm' type.

Membranous structures, mostly described as related to the atrioventricular valves, have been discussed thoroughly in many publications, often in combination with other obstructing influences, which in many cases tend to be abnormal attachments – mostly of mitral valvular tissue – or connections.

What one should always keep in mind is the variation in causes of pulmonary stennsis described by the various authors, which may depend mostly on the period of collecting of the postmortem material. This is another reason why one should be caútious in the interpretation of findings from the literature.

OBSTRUCTION DUE TO MALALIGNMENT

The most frequently described type of left ventricular outflow tract obstruction in transposition with interventricular communication is closely related to a malalignment septal defect, which may result from malorientation of the infundibular septum (fig. 1-4). The infundibular septum is the structure interposing between the semilunar valves (20, 21); in normal hearts it is incorporated on top of the ventricular septum. In these hearts with malalignment ventricular septal defect the so-called anterolateral muscle bundle of the left ventricle may also be involved in the outflow tract obstruction. This is the muscle bundle separating the anterior leaflet of the mitral valve from the anterior border of the left ventricle. It borders on the left semilunar cusp and extends into the anterolateral wall of the left ventricle (fig. 1b, 3b, 4) (22, 23). The anterolateral muscle bundle is found in about 70 percent of heart specimens with transposition as compared with 50 percent of cases in normal hearts (24). Anderson et al. describe this muscle bundle as the ventriculo-infundibular fold of the left ventricle (20).

The first time an obstruction due to malalignment as such was described was by Quero Jiménez et al. in 1973 (6, 14) as a '. . . positional deviation of the conal septum (= infundibular septum) inside the conus (which) resulted in obstructive anomalies of the subpulmonary outflow tract . . .'. They de-

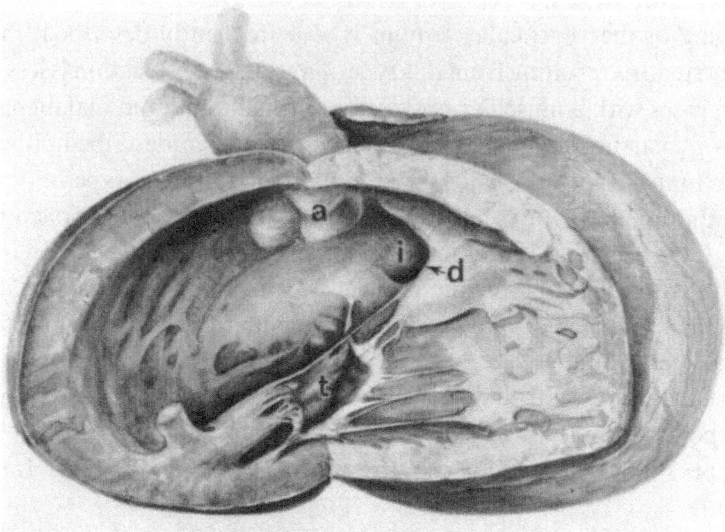

Figure 1a. Right ventricular view of a heart with transposition of the great arteries and malalignment ventricular septal defect (d) with extreme leftward deviation of the infundibular septum (i). The defect is partly bounded by aortic valve tissue and by infundibular septum. a = aortic orifice; t = tricuspid orifice. (By courtesy of the Editor, *Br. Heart J.*, 1978).

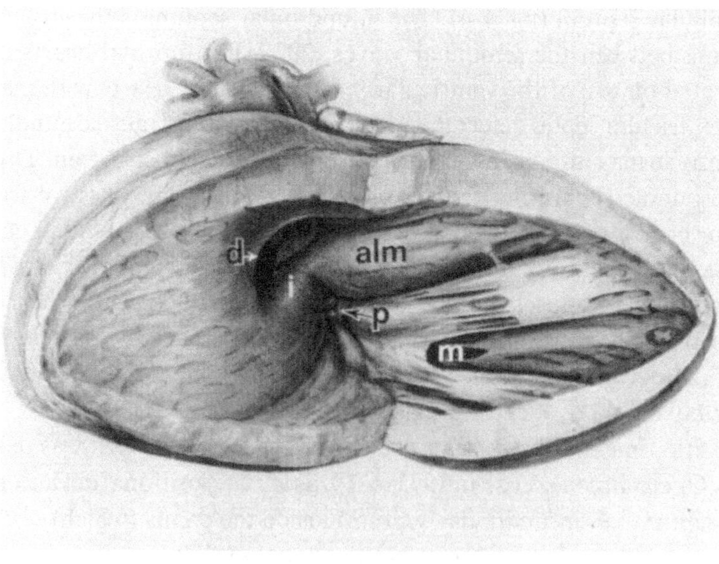

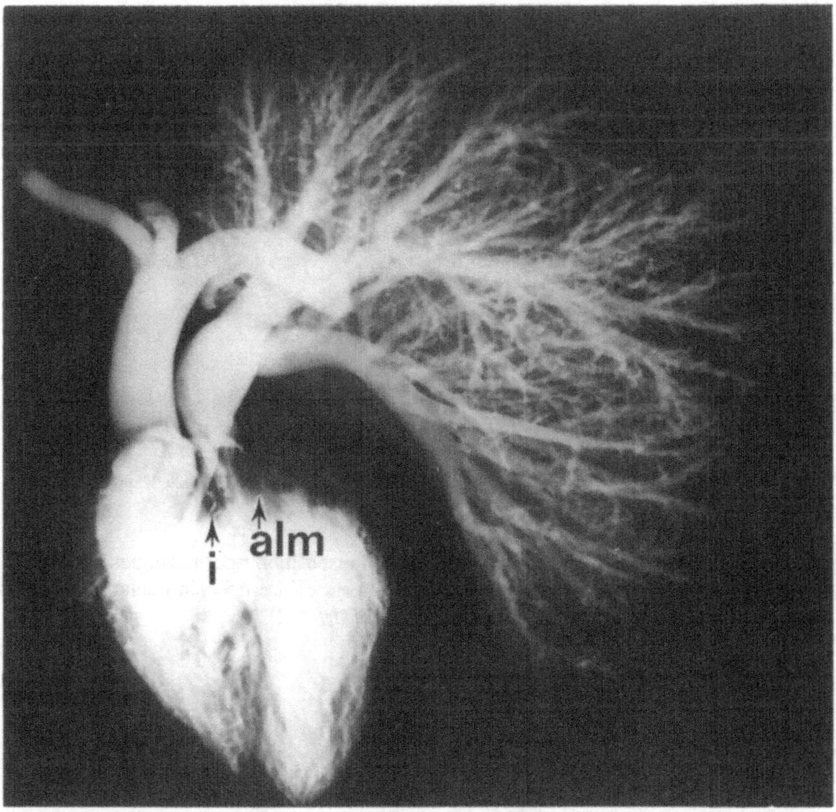

Figure 2. Postmortem X-ray of a heart with transposition and the same type of interventricular communication and subpulmonary obstruction as in figure 1. A severe obstruction of the left ventricular outflow tract by infundibular septum (i) and anterolateral muscle bundle of the left ventricle (alm) is visible.

scribed overriding of the infundibular septum on the ventricular septum as well. In some more recent publications, some of these obstructions in malalignment VSD, though not mentioned, might be present, as judged from the photographs and an interpretation of the anatomical descriptions given (3,

Figure 1b. Left ventricular view of same heart as figure 1a. The obstructive infundibular septum (i) can be seen joining the anterolateral muscle bundle of the left ventricle (alm) which is also obstructing. There is a posterior displacement of the pulmonary orifice (p). m = mitral orifice; d = ventricular septal defect. (By courtesy of the Editor, *Br. Heart J.*, 1978).

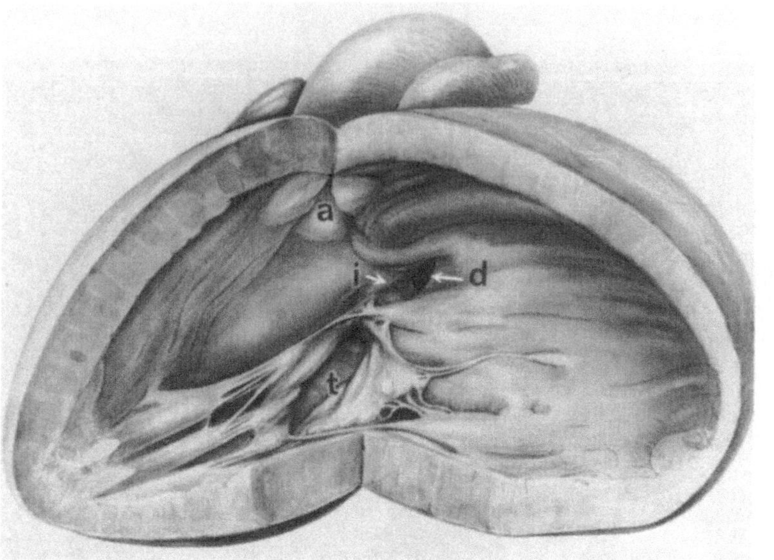

Figure 3a. Right ventricular view of a heart with transposition and malalignment with less extreme deviation of the infundibular septum (i). a = aortic orifice; d = ventricular septal defect; t = tricuspid orifice. (By courtesy of the Editor, *Br. Heart J.*, 1978).

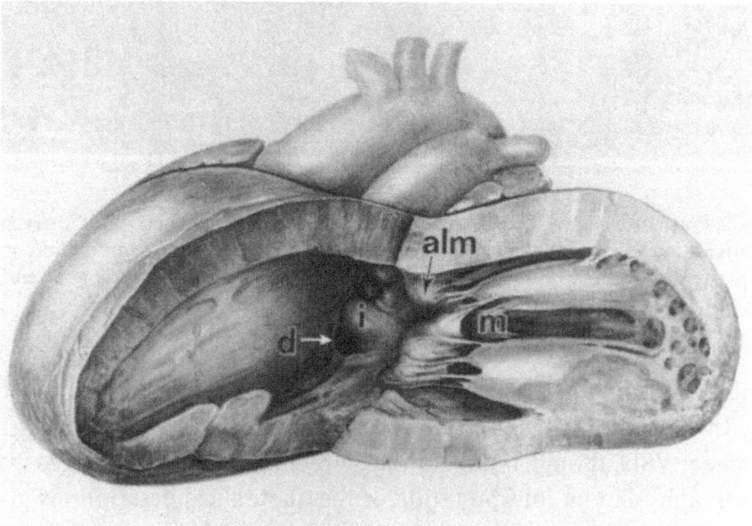

Figure 3b. Left ventricular view of same heart as figure 3a. The obstructing structures, infundibular septum (i) and anterolateral muscle bundle of the left ventricle (alm), are situated at opposite sides of the pulmonary orifice. m = mitral orifice; d = ventricular septal defect. (By courtesy of the Editor, *Br. Heart J.*, 1978).

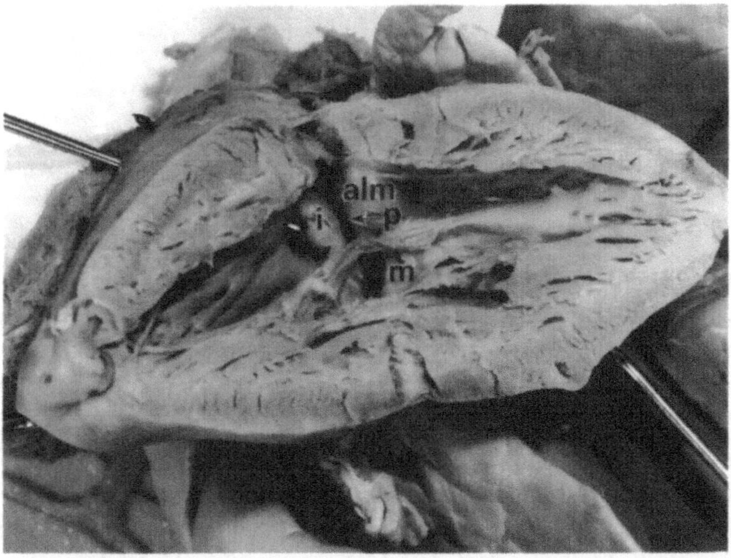

Figure 4. Left ventricular view of a heart with transposition and malalignment septal defect with less extreme deviation of the infundibular septum (i). A probe lies in the defect. Obstructing factors are anterolateral muscle bundle (alm) and infundibular septum at the left and right side of the pulmonary orifice respectively. m = mitral orifice; p = pulmonary orifice.

13, 19). Recently, many cases have been described by Van Praagh (9) and by Quero Jiménez et al. (16), while van Gils et al. (2) proposed a categorization in two types of malalignment defect which they showed to be in close relationship to the type and degree of pulmonary stenosis, although they agree that the number of heart specimens investigated is rather small (11 specimens).

They (2) described that an extreme leftward deviation of the infundibular septum results in a pulmonary stenosis caused by the infundibular septum together with an anterolateral muscle bundle. Both structures met at the anterior side of the pulmonary orifice, which was displaced posteriorly. The ventricular septal defect in the 6 cases thus described was in direct contact with aortic valve cusp tissue, the pulmonary stenosis was mostly severe (fig. 1a, 1b, 2). A less extreme deviation of the infundibular septum in another 5 cases where the infundibular septum separated septal defect and aortic valve, results in a pulmonary stenosis caused by infundibular septum and anterolateral muscle bundle. These structures were separated from each other at the right and at the left side of the pulmonary orifice respectively (fig. 3a, 3b, 4). The stenosis in these last 5 cases was moderate in contrast to the 6 cases first mentioned.

OBSTRUCTION DUE TO BULGING OF THE VENTRICULAR SEPTUM

Somewhat less frequently described in literature is a bulging of the ventricular septum into the cavity of the left ventricle. It is described as a prominence of the septal wall of the left ventricle protruding into its cavity (1-3, 11, 12, 17) and as a markedly hypertrophied mid portion of the ventricular septum (25). Shaher et al. (8) suggested that this type of left ventricular outflow tract obstruction might occur as a hypertrophic reaction resulting from pulmonary valvular or subvalvular stenosis and diminished pulmonary blood flow. Silove and Taylor (26) however point to the possible apposition of the mitral valve on the ventricular septum in transposition, which they think is related to the progressive fibrous endothelial thickening on this side of the septum. This relation is also confirmed in the observations of Bühlmeyer et al. (10), who saw in 15 patients an apposition of the closed mitral valve leaflets to a bulging of the ventricular septum. This relation is also in accordance with the findings of several other investigators (1, 2, 8, 25) who found the bulging mainly or only in the mid part of the septum at the site where an apposition of the mitral valve could be expected.

The pulmonary stenosis resulting from bulging was described as mild to moderate (2, 8).

DIFFUSE SUBVALVULAR FIBROMUSCULAR STENOSIS ('TUNNEL-SHAPED OUTFLOW TRACT')

A narrow tunnel of fibromuscular tissue lined by thickened fibroelastic tissue extends from the stenosed pulmonary valve to the ventricular septal defect below (7, 8, 10-12, 16-18). It is remarkable that in all cases described the distance between septal defect and pulmonary valve was rather large. This would agree with Lev's suggestion, that the subvalvular stenosis in transposition may be acquired because of the distance between the defect and the pulmonary valve, and that the fibroelastic reaction may be attributed to the turbulent blood flow (4). Shaher described this type of obstruction as severe (8, 18).

LOCALIZED SUBVALVULAR FIBROMUSCULAR STENOSIS

A ring of fibrous tissue, immediately below the pulmonary valve, obstructs the outflow tract of the left ventricle, there is often associated pulmonary valvular stenosis (fig. 5) (2, 7-13, 16, 17, 19). According to Shaher (8, 18), the obstruction should be severe; van Gils et al. (2) described 1 case with an associated markedly thickened anterior left ventricular wall and a moderate pulmonary stenosis.

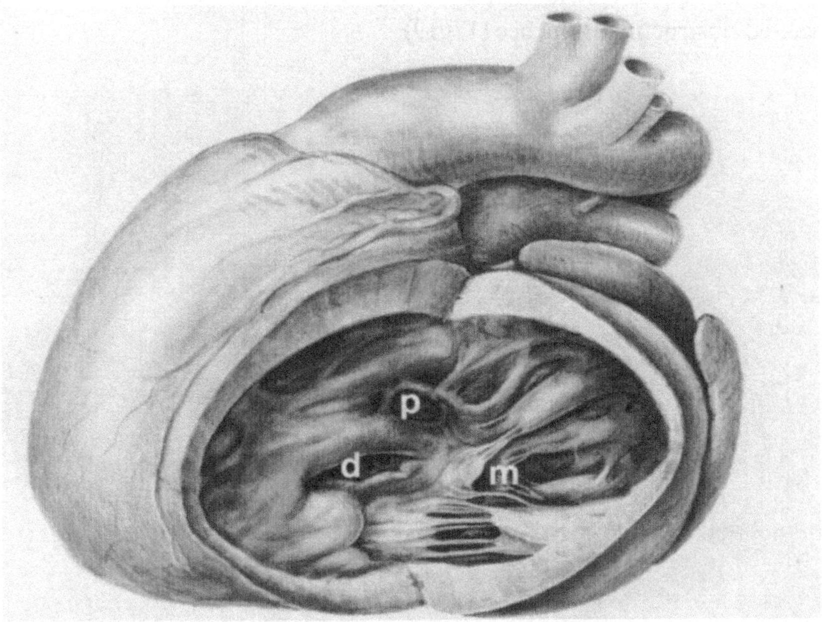

Figure 5. Left ventricular view of a heart with transposition and interventricular communication with a localized subvalvular fibromuscular ring, obstructing the outflow tract. m = mitral orifice; p = pulmonary orifice; d = ventricular septal defect.

OBSTRUCTIONS RELATED TO THE ATRIOVENTRICULAR VALVES

Attention should be paid to a remarkable appearance of the mitral valve, a cleft in the anterior leaflet, which is reported several times in the literature.

This condition was reported in association with valvular pulmonary stenosis once (8) and twice together with malalignment defect (6, 13). Five cases of associated abnormal attachment of the cleft anterior mitral leaflet on the ventricular septum are also described, once with an apparent counterclockwise rotation of the mitral valve (27) and four cases with a deviation to the left of the anterior part of the ventricular septum (fig. 6) (2). An abnormal attachment of the anterior mitral valve leaflet to the ventricular septum was also a rather frequent cause of pulmonary stenosis, several times described as the only cause (6, 10, 16, 19) or with an apparent counterclockwise rotation of the mitral valve apparatus (28), and five times with a cleft mitral valve leaflet (see above). Redundant atrioventricular valvular tissue may also have an associated obstructing influence (17, 19).

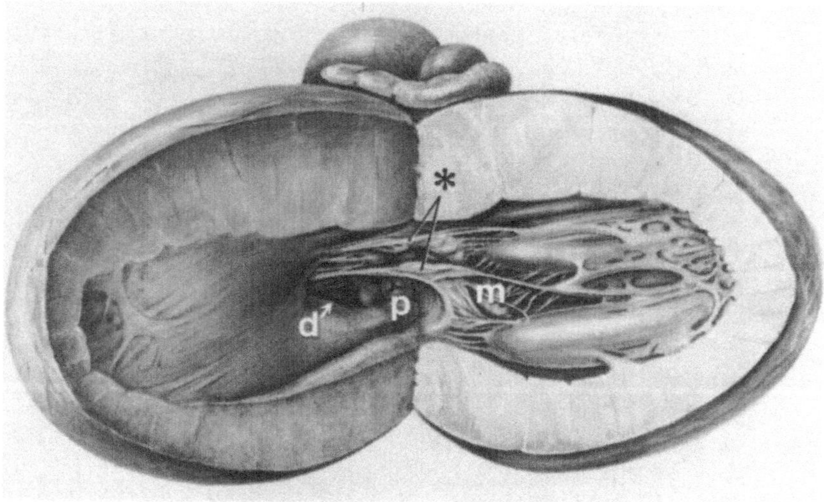

Figure 6. Left ventricular view of a heart with transposition and interventricular communication. The cleft anterior leaflet of the mitral valve is anomalously attached to the anterior part of the ventricular septum, which is deviated to the left. * = both parts of the cleft anterior mitral leaflet; m = mitral orifice; p = pulmonary orifice; d = ventricular septal defect. (By courtesy of the Editor, *Br. Heart J.*, 1978).

Rosenquist et al. (28) made a thorough investigation of the mitral valve in cases of transposition. They also reported mitral valve anomalies in specimens with associated 'subvalvular' pulmonary stenosis, either a restricted free margin of the anterior leaflet or a so poorly developed space between the left ventricular papillary muscles that these appeared fused together.

Elsewhere in this book Wenink (p. 129) reported a '. . . leftsided prominence (which) may be related to a leftward deviation of the anterior portion of the ventricular septum', which occurred mostly as an entity with an abnormal attachment of the cleft mitral valve leaflet on the septum (2). Redundant atrioventricular valvular tissue has been mentioned fairly often as an obstructing factor, mostly in association with many other influences. It may be either mitral valvular tissue (2, 17, 19, 26) – which was in some cases so redundant that it even protruded through the septal defect towards the right ventricle – or tricuspid valvular tissue protruding through the defect (10, 19, 29). Sometimes redundant subvalvular tissue was not categorized within this scheme (17). Attention has to be paid (this chapter, p. 166) to the possible apposition of the mitral valve on the ventricular septum which might have an influence both on the mitral valve and on the (bulging) ventricular septum (10, 26).

REFERENCES

1. Elliott, L. P., Neufeld, H. N., Anderson, R. C., Adams, P. and Edwards, J. E., Complete transposition of the great vessels. I. An anatomic study of sixty cases. *Circulation* 27, 1105 (1963).
2. van Gils, F. A. W., Moulaert, A. J., Oppenheimer-Dekker, A. and Wenink, A. C. G., Transposition of the great arteries with ventricular septal defect and pulmonary stenosis. *Br. Heart J.*, 40. 494 (1978).
3. Imamura, E. S., Morikawa, T., Tatsuno, K., Konno, S., Arai, T. and Sakakibara, S., Surgical considerations of ventricular septal defect associated with complete transposition of the great arteries and pulmonary stenosis with special reference to the Rastelli operation. *Circulation* 44, 914 (1971).
4. Lev, M., Alcalde, V. M. and Baffes, T. G., Pathologic anatomy of complete transposition of the arterial trunks. *Pediatrics* 28, 293 (1961).
5. Paul, M. H., Van Praagh, S. and Van Praagh, R., Transposition of the great arteries. In: *Paediatric Cardiology* (ed. H. Watson), London 1968.
6. Quero-Jiménez, M., Castro Gussoni, M. C., Moreno Granados, F. and Pérez Diaz, L., Transposition des gros vaisseaux. Anatomie pathologique. *Coeur*, Numéro spécial, 4, 177 (1973).
7. Shaher, R. M., *Complete transposition of the great arteries*. Academic Press, New York & London 1973.
8. Shaher, R. M., Puddu, G. C., Khoury, G., Moës, C. A. F. and Mustard, W. T., Complete transposition of the great vessels with anatomic obstruction of the outflow tract of the left ventricle. Surgical implications of anatomic findings. *Am. J. Cardiol.* 19, 658 (1967).
9. Van Praagh, R., Anatomic types of left ventricular outflow tract obstruction in transposition of the great arteries. In: *Abstract Book of the 15th Annual General Meeting of the Association of European Paediatric Cardiologists*, Gent, Belgium, 10, 1977.

10. Bühlmeyer, K., Tacke, E. and Mocellin, R., Angiocardiographic and functional studies in patients with transposition of the great arteries and left ventricular outflow tract obstruction. In: *Abstract Book of the 15th Annual General Meeting of the Association of European Paediatric Cardiologists*, Gent, Belgium, 14, 1977.
11. Daicoff, G. R., Schiebler, G. L., Elliott, L. P., Van Mierop, L. H. S., Bartley, T. D., Gessner, I. H. and Wheat, M. W., Surgical repair of complete transposition of the great arteries with pulmonary stenosis. *Ann. Thor. Surg.* 7, 529 (1969).
12. Fisher, E. H. R., Muster, A. J., Lev, M. and Paul, M. H., Angiocardiographic and anatomic findings in transposition of the great arteries with left ventricular outflow tract gradients. *Am. J. Cardiol.* 25, 95 (1970).
13. Lancelin, B., Pauly-Laubry, C., Guerinon, J., Tricot, J.-L., Bouchard, F. and Maurice, P., Transposition des gros vaisseaux avec sténose pulmonaire et communication interventriculaire. Aspect anatomique et chirurgical à propos de 10 observations. *Arch. Mal. Coeur* 68, 339 (1975).
14. Quero-Jiménez, M. and Pérez Martínez, V., Uncommon conal pathology in complete dextrotransposition of the great arteries with ventricular septal defect. *Chest* 66, 411 (1974).
15. Quero-Jiménez, M., Casanova Gómez, M. and Burgueros Valero, M., Tipos de communicación interventricular en la dextrotransposición completa de las grandes arterias. *Rev. esp. Cardiol.* 28, 469 (1975).
16. Quero-Jiménez, M., Casanova Gómez, M., Marsico, F., Quero-Jiménez, C., Calabró, R. and Burgueros Valero, M., Morphologic aspects of the left ventricular outflow tract in transposition of the great arteries. In: *Abstract Book of the 15th Annual General Meeting of the Association of European Paediatric Cardiologists*, Gent, Belgium, 11, 1977.
17. Rastelli, G. C., Wallace, R. B. and Ongley, P. A., Complete repair of transposition of the great arteries with pulmonary stenosis. A review and report of a case corrected by using a new surgical technique. *Circulation* 39, 83 (1969).
18. Shaher, R. M., Moës, C. A. F. and Khoury, G., Radiologic and angiocardiographic findings in complete transposition of the great vessels with left ventricular outflow tract obstruction. *Radiology* 88, 1092 (1967).
19. Shrivastava, S., Tadavarthy, S. M., Fukuda, T. and Edwards, J. E., Anatomic causes of pulmonary stenosis in complete transposition. *Circulation* 54, 154 (1976).
20. Anderson, R. H., Becker, A. E. and Van Mierop, L. H. S., What should we call the 'crista'? *Br. Heart J.* 39. 856 (1977).
21. Lev, M., The conotruncus: I. Its normal inversion and conus absorption. *Circulation* 46, 634 (1972).
22. Moulaert, A. J., *Ventricular septal defects and anomalies of the aortic arch.* Thesis, Leiden, 1974.
23. Moulaert, A. J. and Oppenheimer-Dekker, A., Anterolateral muscle bundle of the left ventricle, bulboventricular flange and subaortic stenosis. *Am. J. Cardiol.* 37, 78 (1976).
24. Oppenheimer-Dekker, A., Wenink, A. C. G., van Gils, F. A. W., Gittenberger-de Groot, A. C. and Moulaert, A. J., Transposition of the great arteries: morphological study of 150 cases. *J. Anat.* 122, 724 (1976).
25. Mehrizi, A., Rowe, R. D., Hutchins, G. M. and Folger, G. M., Transposition of the great vessels with pulmonary stenosis and ventricular seppta seppa septal defect. *Bull. Johns Hopk. Hosp.* 119, 200 (1966).
26. Silove, E. D. and Taylor, J. F. N., Angiographic and anatomical features of subvalvular left ventricular outflow obstruction in transposition of the great arteries. The possible role of the anterior mitral valve leaflet *Pediatr. Radiol.* 1, 87 (1973).
27. Layman, T. E. and Edwards, J. E., Anomalies of the cardiac valves associated with complete transposition of the great vessels. *Am. J. Cardiol.* 19, 247 (1967).

28. Rosenquist, G. C., Stark, J. and Taylor, J. F. N., Congenital mitral valve disease in transposition of the great arteries. *Circulation* 51, 731 (1975).
29. Riemenschneider, T. A., Goldberg, S. J., Ruttenberg, H. D. and Gyepes, M. T., Subpulmonic obstruction in complete (d) transposition produced by redundant tricuspid tissue. *Circulation* 39, 603 49).

PART II

TRANSPOSITION OF THE GREAT ARTERIES

C. Clinical aspects

16. THE SURGICAL TREATMENT OF TRANSPOSITION OF THE GREAT ARTERIES

A. G. BROM AND J. M. J. DE LEERSNIJDER

HISTORY

The surgical management of transposition of the great arteries started in 1950 by creating an atrial septal defect to increase mixing between the two circulations as reported by Blalock and Hanlon.

The attempts of Mustard and Bailey in 1952 to reverse the transposed great arteries directly were unsuccessfull.

In 1953 Lillehei and Varco transferred the right pulmonary veins to the right atrium and the inferior vena cava to the left atrium, and so they introduced a partially physiologic correction. The concept of rearrangement of venous flow within the atria was proposed by Albert in 1955 on the basis of animal experiments. Merendino in 1957 attempted intra-atrial diversionary procedures by using a prosthetic sponge.

It was Åke Senning of Stockholm who on June 10th, 1958 reported success in transposing the atria in a 9 year old boy.

The method of Mustard described in 1964 using pericardium for redirecting venous flow within the atria had received wide use and good results.

Rastelli at the Mayo-clinic (1969) developed a technique allowing the left ventricle to be connected to the aorta and the right ventricle to the pulmonary artery using a conduit which contained a valve.

More recently Jatene et al. reported successfull anatomic correction of transposition of the great arteries by transposing the great arteries and reattaching the coronaries.

PALLIATIVE PROCEDURES

Most patients with transposition of the great arteries have severe cyanosis which appears in the first days of life. Once the clinical diagnosis is suspected, cardiac catheterisation should be undertaken and if diagnosis of transposition is confirmed a balloon septostomy (Rashkind and Miller) should be performed. A balloon-tipped catheter is advanced into the right atrium and through the foramen ovale into the left atrium. The balloon is inflated with contrast material and then pulled forcibly through the foramen ovale enlarging or tearing the atrium septum.

In some cases other palliative treatment beside the balloon septostomy is required, but this is usually the case only in infants under six months of age.

1.1 In the presence of a large ventricular septal defect, banding can be necessary. The main pulmonary artery is narrowed to about one third its original size by a constricting band, to limit pulmonary blood flow and prevent pulmonary hypertension.

1.2 In the case of a ventricular septal defect with severe pulmonary stenosis it may be necessary to establish a pulmonary-aorta shunt in order to improve the child's general condition. The Blalock-Taussig shunt (subclavian-pulmonary arteries anastomosis) and Waterston shunt (anastomosis between ascending aorta and right pulmonary artery) are preferred.

1.3 When balloon septostomy is unsuccessfull or insufficient (pressure gradient between left and right atrium) the atrial septum is for most part resected (Blalock-Hanlon operation).

CORRECTIVE OPERATIONS

These are divided into two groups, which may be classified as follows: 2.1 In operations of the first group, aorta and pulmonary artery are anastomosed to the appropriate ventricle, i.e. the aorta to the left and the pulmonary artery to the right. These operations can generally be performed only if the pressure in the left ventricle is sufficiently high for the systemic circulation.

A. In patients with pulmonary stenosis and a large, favourably localized VSD, the latter can be so closed that the aorta corresponds with the left ventricle. After occlusion of the proximal pulmonary artery, a homograft or plastic prosthesis (with valve) is used to establish an anastomosis between right ventricle and pulmonary artery (Rastelli procedure). The same can be done in the case of VSD and banding of the pulmonary artery.

B. A much more interesting possibility is the one devised by Baffes and first performed by Jatene. In the infant, both coronary arteries are transposed to the pulmonary artery behind them. Aorta and pulmonary artery are then cut (distal to the implanted coronary arteries) and the distal ends of the vessels are decussated and sutured to the proximal ends. This creates a normal situation: aorta with coronary vessels from the left, and pulmonary artery from the right.

The operation can only be performed if the pressure in the left ventricle is sufficiently high or if this ventricle still has the capacity to build up a higher systemic pressure immediately after the operation (Lover's patient). The operation cannot be performed in the presence of a severe pulmonary stenosis.

A disadvantage is that reconstruction of the pulmonary artery often calls for the use of a plastic prosthesis, and this poses problems in these small patients. Several successfull operations have been described (Ross, Yacoub), but the mortality is still high.

C. The Stansel procedure is a variant of the previous two procedures. We are informed that this type of operation is performed in some clinics with success. A different approach is done by Dr. Aubert from Marseille. His operation consists of a switch without transplantation of the coronary artery.

In the second group of operations

2.2 The correction is effected by reversing not the arterial but the venous pole. The blood from the venae cavae is guided to the left ventricle and thence to the pulmonary artery. The blood from the pulmonary veins is guided to the aorta via the right ventricle.

A. The best known operation is the Mustard procedure. After resection of the entire atrial septum, a patch is placed in the atria so that reversal is effected. Modifications have been introduced to avoid two post-operative complications: (1) dysrhythmias and (2) obstructions to flow from the venae cavae or the pulmonary veins. The widespread use of the Mustard operation increased knowledge of intra-cardiac conduction: The sinus node, its artery or the atrioventricular node. Damage may result in sudden death even some years after operation. The risk of stenosis of the venae cavae and the lung veins can be avoided by careful measuring and cutting the patch to the correct shape.

B. In addition to the Mustard procedure there is the Senning operation, successfully performed before the Mustard procedure was introduced but relegated to the background in recent years. In this operation the venous reversal is effected with the aid of the remnants of atrial septum, partly in and partly outside the heart. Like the Mustard procedure this operation can cause lesions of the conduction system. Otherwise the amount of foreign material used is very small.

DISCUSSION

1. If the anatomy and physiology are favourable and if the mortality decreases with increasing experience, then arterial reversal according to Anagnastopoulos and Jatene is undoubtedly the operation of choice. We have assumed that the systolic pressure on the coronary arteries will not prematurely affect these vessels.
2. A Rastelli procedure can be carried out in some patients with transposition (favourably localized, large ventricular septal defect and pulmonary stenosis or banding). As a rule, however, this is not feasible until after the second year of life (in view of the space required in the thoracic cavity for the large prosthesis).
3. In view of the very low mortality of venous reversal, these operations are to be preferred. The major problem in these cases, however is: will the right ventricle and the tricuspid valve tolerate the systemic pressure over a period of about 70 years?

It is difficult to decide between the Mustard and the Senning procedure. The differences between the two procedures are as follows:

1. A large patch is used in the Mustard and a very small one in the Senning procedure. We are not yet certain of what will happen with the fairly large prosthesis in the heart as these children treated in infancy, grow to adulthood. An advantage of the Senning operation is that normal growth of the tissues used takes place.
2. Even if we assume that atrial function is far less important than ventricular function in maintaining cardiac output, we must consider which atria contract better, those which contract against a stiff, immobile prosthesis as in the Mustard procedure or those in which the new right atrium contracts normally while the left contracts against a yielding right atrium as in the Senning procedure.
3. In the Mustard procedure the size of the intra-atrial baffle has to be determined with great accuracy lest it be too large (causing obstruction of the pulmonary veins) or too small (causing stenosis of the superior vena cava or the new right atrium). In the Senning operation this problem is eliminated because the heart itself determines the size of the baffle.

CONCLUSION

We believe that the Senning operation affords a more logical solution to the problem of venous reversal and it became – outside those cases where arterial switch is possible – the treatment of choice in Transposition of the Great Arteries in our department.

The decision to revert to the Senning procedure was influenced by (1) the good haemodynamic condition of two patients operated by this method in 1962 and 1963, and otherwise (2) the apply of the principles of the Senning operation (trapeziform roof over the pulmonary veins and two channels for the venae cavae) to the Mustard procedure.

From December 1975 to September 1977, 30 patients were treated by the Senning procedure. There were 22 males and 8 females. The weights of our patients at the time of operation varied from 4.5 kg to 16 kg, their ages from 4 months to 3½ years. All patients were in sinus rhythm at the time of operation.

Two patients died. The 28 surviving patients have been followed for periods ranging from a few weeks to well over a year. All patients are greatly improved with disappearance of cyanosis and fatigue. 24 are in sinus rhythm, and 4 have junctional rhythm. Few weeks after operation cardiac catheterisation was carried out in all patients, except four. Mean pressure differences between venae cavae and new right atrium did not exceed 4 mmHg.

In our hands the mortality of Sennings operation is approximately the same as that of Mustards operation. The incidence of junctional rhythm in the survivors seems to be slightly less after the Senning procedure and the improvement in the condition of the patients is striking after either operation.

In the first period of this 'revival' one was reluctant to use the Senning procedure during the first months of life. Experience gained since, has convinced us that particularly for these small infants the Senning procedure is indicated. Our opinion is endorsed by the policy in several important cardiac centers in the world to perform the Senning procedure in those cases, in which for anatomical or physiological reasons an arterial switch is impossible.

17. ARRHYTHMIAS FOLLOWING MUSTARD'S OPERATION FOR TRANSPOSITION OF THE GREAT ARTERIES

M. J. TYNAN

The first report of arrhythmias occurring as a consequence of Mustard's operations for transposition of the great arteries (ventriculo-arterial discordance with atrio-ventricular concordance) was in 1965 (1). Twelve years later we are still uncertain of the frequency with which these complications occur and of the mechanism of their production. It is a particularly appropriate time to review our understanding of this problem because the occurrence of arrhythmias, amongst other complications, has been cited as a reason for preferring the newly introduced arterial swith operation (2) for the definitive treatment of transposition.

TYPES OF ARRHYTHMIA AND THEIR INCIDENCE

Following the operation, the majority of patients exhibit a decrease in the amplitude of the P wave but maintain a normal P wave axis (3-6). Since this is not strictly an arrhythmia, patients with this finding alone may be considered to be in sinus rhythm. It is probable that the change in P wave amplitude is due to a minor damage to the sinu-atrial node but that the pacemaker still remains within the node.

Definite arrhythmias which are a consequence of the operation include sinu-atrial block, first described by Zuberbuhler and Bauersfeld (7), the tachycardia-bradycardia syndrome (6, 7), atrial flutter (1, 3, 4, 6, 8, 11), atrial fibrillation (9), paroxysmal supraventricular tachycardia (4, 8), junctional rhythm (4, 6, 8, 10, 11, 12), atrio-ventricular dissociation and heart block (4, 12), wandering pacemaker and coronary sinus rhythm (4, 5, 7, 9, 10) and in one case ventricular tachycardia (9). The different types of rhythm and conduction disturbances occur with differing frequency in the different series. Tachyarrhythmias have been reported in 20% to 36% of patients in some series (4, 6, 7) but none of the 47 patients in the series of Clarkson et al. (5) had such arrhythmias. Similarly, the overall incidence of arrhythmias varies from

Table 1. Number of patients in sinus rhythm at late follow up after Mustard's operation.

	Total	No. in S.R.	% in S.R.
El Said et al. (4)*	27	10	37
Greenwood et al. (7)	35	12	34
Aberdeen (11)	112	63	65
Clarkson et al. (5)	46	40	87
Lewis et al. (6)	110	32	29

Key: S.R. = sinus rhythm
* Follow up at 6 weeks to one year

series to series. In table 1 are shown the results abstracted from five reports. The percentage of patients found to be in sinus rhythm varies from 29% to 87%. However, the methodology of the studies has a profound effect on the results observed. In their report El-Said (4) and his colleagues made two major points: firstly, patients in sinus rhythm at a given examination may be observed at other times to have arrhythmias and secondly, the number of patients in sinus rhythm declined with increasing time after surgery. Thus, at 6 weeks to 1 year after surgery, 37% were in sinus rhythm, whilst at 1 to 3 year follow up, only 17% were. Taking these two factors into account, El-Said et al. found that only 25% of their patients were consistently in sinus rhythm post-operatively. In table 2 are presented the results of four series (4, 5, 11) showing the numbers of patients never to have been in other than sinus rhythm. Included in the final figure are transient post-operative arrhythmias because it is known from other conditions that transient post-operative arrhythmias are not necessarily benign in the long term (13) and thus even after an apparent return to sinus rhythm, these arrhythmias cannot be ignored. Even when transient post-operative arrhythmias are included, the incidence of these complications is still probably underestimated. In a recent study (14) using 24-hour tape monitoring of the ECG on 21 survivors of Mustard's operation,

Table 2. Number of patients never in other than sinus rhythm.

	Total	No. in S.R.	% in S.R.
El-Said et al. (4)	60	3	5
Aberdeen et al. (11)	112	57	51
Clarkson et al. (5)	46	36	78
Lewis et al. (6)	110	26	24

4 of the 14 patients thought to be in sinus rhythm were found to have significant arrhythmias. Thus, in this series, the apparent incidence of arrhythmias was 6 in 21, i.e. 21%, but the true incidence was 10 in 21 or 48%.

The differences in results from different centres using different protocols to study the problem, make it impossible to give an accurate estimate of the frequency with which arrhythmias occur. All that can be said is that they appear to affect a significant number of patients, probably between 20% and 50% of the survivors. Furthermore, one important feature does emerge. The heart's rhythm after Mustard's operation is not a static phenomenon, it varies from time to time during the day and it changes with the length of time elapsing after surgery.

MECHANISMS OF PRODUCTION OF ARRHYTHMIAS AFTER MUSTARD'S OPERATION

Sinu-atrial node damage

Damage to the sinu-atrial (S.A.) node may be inferred from the alteration in P wave morphology described above. However, more serious damage is probably the cause of the tachycardia-bradycardia syy syndrome, sinu-atrial block and a sinus arrest. Using a long-term tape monitoring of the ECG Greenwood et al. (8) found five of 35 patients to be suffering from the sick sinus syndrome after Mustard's operation. This type of investigation is useful not only for the detection of arrhythmias, but also for assessing their severity and probable cause. Figure 1 shows one of several episodes of asystole observed during a 24-hour period in a patient known to have episodes of paroxysmal tachycar-

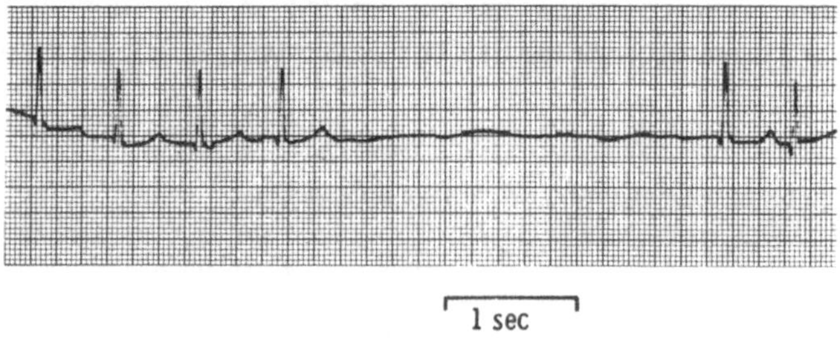

Figure 1. A recording of part of a 24 hour tape recording of the ECG in a patient known to have had paroxysmal tachycardia after Mustard's operation. Several similar gaps of three seconds or more were observed. These findings strongly suggest sinu-atrial node damage.

dia and syncope. This finding strongly suggests that the arrhythmias were due to S.A. node damage. As further evidence that S.A. node injury is an important cause of arrhythmias due to Mustard's operation, Gillette et al. (15) found prolonged sinus node recovery times in 4 of 9 patients studied. In 2 of these the junctional area recovered before the sinus node. Whilst, in addition, El-Said et al. (4) observed pathological evidence of damage to the sinu-atrial node in 2 patients dying in the immediate post-operative period and in 3 patients dying later. In the early deaths, haemorrhage into the sinus node was the main feature, but in those dying later, the node appeared to have been completely destroyed. Thus, without doubt, S.A. node damage is an important cause of arrhythmias after Mustard's operation.

Atrio-ventricular node and penetrating bundle damage
Atrio-ventricular (A.V.) node damage accounts for those cases demonstrating atrio-ventricular Wenckebach and may explain some cases of heart block, the remaining cases of heart block being due to damage to the bundle of His. In general, it is only in situations where the standard ECG or 24-hour tape suggests A.V. nodal or His bundle damage that intracardiac electrophysiological studies demonstrate an abnormality (9, 14). There is little controversy about methods of avoiding atrio-ventricular conduction problems since the anatomy of the A.V. node and the bundle of His is well known and can, if need be, be demonstrated during operation (16).

DISTURBANCES OF INTRA-ATRIAL CONDUCTION

Although some arrhythmias can only be explained on the basis of damage to the S.A. or A.V. nodes or to damage to the atrio-ventricular conduction system, there are others for which alternative explanations are possible. Junctional rhythm may be an escape rhythm following damage to the sinu-atrial node but delayed internodal conduction has been suggested as an alternative cause (8, 17). Similarly, atrial flutter, which may be a re-entry phenomenon, has been attributed to damage to the 'internodal tracts' (11, 17).

The evidence relating to internodal conduction delay as a cause of arrhythmias after Mustard's operation is conflicting. On the one hand Wittig et al. (18) in an intra-operative mapping study demonstrated conduction delay in the posterior atrio-ventricular nodal input when the incision crossed the crista terminalis or when coronary sinus cutback was used. This was not associated with abnormal internodal conduction unless there was concomitant damage

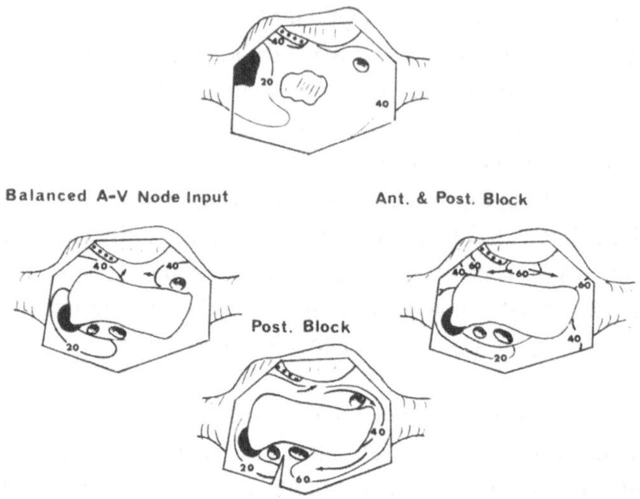

Figure 2. This figure is based on the observations of Wittig et al. (1977). The upper center panel shows atrial activation following a longitudinal atriotomy not extending across the sulcus terminalis. The stippled area is the atrio-ventricular bundle. The isochorous lines are labelled in m. sec. Balanced A-V node input is seen after patch insertion with a normal sequence of atrial and A-V nodal activation. Posterior block due to a lateral atriotomy, however the A-V nodal area is activated normally via the anterior septal route. Anterior and posterior block occurring with a coronary sinus cut back. Both anterior and posterior routes of conduction are delayed sufficiently to allow junctional escape. In all three instances the site of earliest activation of the atria (in black) has moved caudally after the suture of the patch indicating sinu-atrial node damage.

to the anterior atrio-ventricular nodal input. When both inputs were damaged junctional escape was possible (fig. 2). In contrast, Mohri et al. (19) showed experimentally in dogs that circumferential incision of the right atrium and atrial septum was associated, after resuture, with only a temporary prolongation of the P-R interval. All animals being in sinus rhythm with normal P-R intervals by 13-14 weeks after the experiment. Taguchi et al. (20) both in experimental animals and in seven children, demonstrated that circumferential incision of both atria and transection of the atrial septum, did not result in serious arrhythmias, provided approximately one-sixth of the right atrial and one-third of the left atrial walls remained intact.

CORRELATIONS OF SURGICAL TECHNIQUES WITH ECG FINDINGS

Once more, a somewhat confusing picture emerges. Ebert et al. (11) suggested that the use of coronary sinus cut-back to the left atrium was associated with a high incidence of atrial flutter, while Clarkson et al. (5) observed no tachy arrhythmias in 25 patients who had had this procedure. Other authors (6, 12, 17) have related a diminution in the frequency of arrhythmias to techniques aimed at preservation of 'inter-nodal conducting tracts' and at avoidance of S.A. and A.V. node damage. However, even with these improvements, Lewis et al. (17) reported only 26% of patients to be continuously in sinus rhythm. These authors agree (6, 12, 17) that much of the improvement in results could be due to less frequent damage to the nodes and atrio-ventricular conducting system rather than to preservation of internodal routes of conduction.

RELEVANT OBSERVATIONS IN OTHER CONDITIONS

Surgical interventions other than the Mustard operation, are known to be associated with the development of arrhythmias. Tung et al. (21) observed S.A. node damage in autopsy specimens of patients dying after a variety of open heart operations. In this series there was a high incidence of post-operative tachy-arrhythmias. Similar tachy-arrhythmias have been observed after closure of atrial septal defects (22-24) and correction of the tetralogy of Fallot (8). Clinical and electrophysiological evidence of S.A. node damage has been reported after both atrial septal defect closure (25) and correction of the tetralogy of Fallot (26). In the context of correction of atrial septal defects, sinus node disease appears to be more frequent, both before and after operation in sinus venosus defects than in regular secundum defects (25). Perhaps in the sinus venosus defect the S.A. node is intrinsically more susceptible to damage, but certainly, in this type of defect, the node is more directly at risk during corrective surgery.

Finally, there is some evidence to suggest that atrial fibrillation and flutter of non-surgical origin are associated with a combination of sinus node disease and intra-atrial pathology. Davis and Pomerance (27) noted loss of cells in the sinu-atrial node and fibrosis in the atria in patients with long-standing atrial flutter or fibrillation. There is, however, no unanimity concerning the role of sinu-atrial node disease in this situation since others have observed normal cellularity of the sinus node in similar circumstances (28).

THE CAUSES AND PREVENTION OF ARRHYTHMIAS DUE TO MUSTARD'S OPERATION

Undoubtedly, surgical damage to the S.A. node, the A.V. node or atrio-ventricular conducting system, will lead to arrhythmias. However, it is difficult to understand how a conduction delay in the atria can, by itself, cause rhythm disturbances. A delay of the duration observed by Wittig et al. (18) should cause a transient junctional escape, but if sinus node automaticity and sinu-atrial conduction are not impaired, sinus capture of the junctional focus will occur and subsequently the A-V node will respond normally to the train of impulses received from the S-A node, irrespective of the intra-atrial conduction delay. Even though a conduction delay alone will not lead to a tachy-arrhythmia or brady-arrhythmia, it does provide one of the necessary conditions for the establishment of a re-entry circuit. If the other conditions are fulfilled, atrial tachy-arrhythmias may occur with or without damage to the sinu-atrial node. Any atrial incision or suture line could constitute the anatomical basis for such a circuit. In fact, the patch used in Mustard's operation provides injuries which have topographical similarities to those used by Rosenblueth and Garcia Ramos (29) to initiate experimental atrial flutter-fibrillation. Even in the absence of a large perimeter for a circus movement, micro re-entry circuits in the atria have been demonstrated experimentally (30) and may exist after Mustard's operation. We can conclude that conduction delay in a part of the atria, should not, by itself, lead to arrhythmias. If the S-A node and the A-V node are connected by atrial myocardium, the S.A. node will continue to control the heart rate, perhaps with some prolongation of the P-R interval. In addition to the mechanisms already suggested, disordered automaticity, which has been demonstrated as a temporary post-operative phenomenon (31), may contribute to the causes of tachy-arrhythmias. It is probable that re-entry and disordered automaticity become more evident when the sinus node function is impaired or when the ectopic focus is isolated from its control.

It is obvious that preservation of the sinus node is of prime importance in the prevention of arrhythmias after Mustard's operation (32). The data of Wittig et al. (18) suggest that sinus node injury occurs more frequently than we would have thought and it may be that the altered P wave morphology observed on post-operative ECGs reflects this type of injury. Thus great care must be taken to avoid the node. Cannulation should be performed well away from the junction of the superior vena cava with the right atrium, also the baffle suture line should be carried well away from the S.A. node. The A.V.

node is easy to avoid since its landmarks, the triangle of Koch, are easily identifiable, whilst the atrio-ventricular conduction system can be identified, if need be, by intra-operative mapping studies. Avoidance of re-entry arrhythmias secondary to extensive intra-atrial surgery is much more difficult. In some ways it would be easier if specialised inter-nodal pathways did exist and damage to them was responsible for arrhythmias. However they do not. The suture lines are dictated by the anatomy and incisions such as lateral atriotomy and coronary sinus cut back are made necessary by haemodynamic considerations. It does, however, appear logical to preserve, as far as possible, one direct route – the anterior one – between the S.A. and A.V. nodes since although conduction delay per se does not cause arrhythmia facilitation of S.A. node to A.V. node conduction may help in maintaining sinus rhythm.

Even when all these precautions are observed, arrhythmias will continue to occur as a consequence of Mustard's operation (6, 32). Any measures aimed at further reducing the incidence of arrhythmias due to this or other types of cardiac surgery, must be rigorously evaluated using intraoperative mapping studies, long term tape monitoring and, where indicated, post-operative intracardiac electrophysiological investigations. In this way, we may be able to answer the many questions remaining regarding the incidence, mechanisms of production and prevention of post-operative disturbances of cardiac rhythm.

REFERENCES

1. Aberdeen, E., Waterston, D. J., Carr, I., Graham, G., Bonham Carter, R. E., Subramanian, S., Successful 'correction' of transposed great arteries by Mustard's operation. *Lancet* I, 1233 (1965).
2. Yacoub, M. H., Radley-Smith, R., Hilton, C. J., Anatomical correction of complete transposition of the great arteries and ventricular septal defect. *Br. Med. J.* 1, 1112 (1976).
3. Khoury, G. H., Shaher, R. M., Fowler, R. S., Keith, J. D., Pre-operative and post-operative electrocardiogram in complete transposition of the great vessels. *Am. Heart J.* 72, 199 (1966).
4. El-Said, G., Rosenberg, H. S., Mullins, C. E., Hallman, G. L., Cooley, D. A., McNamara, D. G., Dysrhythmias after Mustard's operation for transposition of the great arteries. *Am. J. Cardiol.* 30, 526 (1972).
5. Clarkson, P. M., Barratt-Boyes, B. G., Neutze, J. M., Late dysrhythmias and disturbances of conduction following Mustard's operation for complete transposition of great arteries. *Circulation* 53, 519 (1976).
6. Lewis, A. B., Lindesmith, G. G., Takahashi, M., Stanton, R. E., Tucker, B. L., Stiles, Q. R., Meyer, B. W., Cardiac rhythm following the Mustard procedure for transposition of the great vessels. *J. Thorac. Cardiovasc. Surg.* 73, 919 (1977).
7. Zuberbuhler, J. R., Bauersfeld, S. R., Unusual arrhythmias after corrective surgery for transposition of the great vessels. *Am. Heart J.* 73, 752 (1967).

8. Greenwood, R. D., Rosenthal, A., Sloss, L. J., LaCorte, M., Nadas, A. S., Sick sinus syndrome after open heart surgery for congenital heart disease. *Circulation* 52, 208 (1975).
9. Isaacson, R., Titus, J. L., Meredith, J., Feldt, R. H., McGoon, D. C., Apparent interruption of atrial conduction pathways after surgical repair of transposition of great arteries. *Am. J. Cardiol.* 30, 533 (1972).
10. Rodriguez-Fernandez, H. L., Kelly, D. T., Collado, A., Haller, J. A., Krovetz, L. J., Rowe, R. D., Haemodynamic data and angiographic findings after Mustard repair for complete transposition of the great arteries. *Circulation* 46, 799 (1972).
11. Ebert, P. A., Gay, W. A., Engle, M. A., Correction of transposition of the great arteries. *Ann. Surg.* 180, 433 (1974).
12. Aberdeen, E., Correction of uncomplicated cases of transposition of the great arteries. *Br. Heart J.* 33, Supplement, 66 (1971).
13. Godman, M. J., Roberts, N. K., Izukawa, T., Late postoperative conduction disturbances after repair of ventricular septal defect and tetralogy of Fallot. *Circulation* 49, 214 (1974).
14. Tynan, M., Reid, D., Goodwin, A., Arrhythmias after Mustard's operation. A 24-hour tape monitoring study. In: Longmore, D. (ed.), *Modern Cardiac Surgery*. Medical and Technical Press. London, in press.
15. Gillette, P. C., El-Said, G. M., Sivarajan, N., Mullins, C. E., Williams, R. L., McNamara, D. G., Electrophysiological abnormalities after Mustard's operation for transposition of the great arteries. *Br. Heart J.* 36, 186 (1974).
16. Waldo, A. L., Krongrad, E., Bowman, F. O., Kaiser, G. A., Husson, G. S., Malm, J. R., Electrophysical considerations during total repair of transposition of the great vessels. *Circulation* 45 & 46, Supplement II, II 34 (1972).
17. Aberdeen, E., Transposition of the great arteries. In: Sabiston, D. C., Spencer, F. C. (ed.) *Gibbon's Surgery of the Chest*. Philadelphia, 1976.
18. Wittig, J. H., DeLaval, M. R., Stark, J., Intraoperative mapping of atrial activation before, during and after the Mustard operation. *J. Thorac. Cardiovasc. Surg.* 73, 1 (1977).
19. Mohri, H., Shigekazu, S., Yates, W. G., Vanini, V., Dillard, D. H., Merendino, K. A., Internodal conduction. *J. Thorac. Cardiovasc. Surg.* 69, 615 (1975).
20. Taguchi, K., Matsumura, H., Hirado, M., Kato, K., A new approach to total repair of transposition of the great vessels. *J. Thorac. Cardiovasc. Surg.* 70, 282 (1977).
21. Tung, K. S. K., James, T. N., Effler, D. B., McCormack, J. L., Injury to the sinus node in open heart operations. *J. Thorac. Cardiovasc. Surg.* 55, 814 (1976).
22. Linde, L. M., Goldberg, S. J., Seigal, S., The natural history of arrhythmias following septal defect repair. *J. Thorac. Cardiovasc. Surg.* 48, 303 (1964).
23. Hawe, A., Rastelli, G. C., Brandenburg, R. O., McGoon, D. C., Embolic complications following repair of atrial septal defect. *Circulation* 39 & 40, Supplement I, I-185 (1969).
24. Cohn, L. H., Morrow, A. G., Braunwald, E., Operative treatment of atrial septal defect: clinical and haemodynamic assessment in 175 patients. *Br. Heart J.* 39, 725 (1967).
25. Clark, E. B., Roland, J. M. A., Vargese, P. J., Neil, C. A., Haller, J. A., Should the sinus venosus A.S.D. be closed? A review of the atrial conduction defects and surgical results in twenty-eight children. *Am. J. Cardiol.* 35, 127 (1975).
26. Niederhauser, H., Simonin, P., Friedli, B., Sinus node function and conduction system after complete repair of tetralogy of Fallot. *Circulation* 52, 214 (1975).
27. Davies, M. J., Pomerance, A., Pathology of atrial fibrillation in man. *Br. Heart J.* 34, 520 (1972).
28. Thery, C., Gosselin, B., Lekieffre, J., Warembourg, H., Pathology of sinoatrial node: Correlations with electrocardiographic findings in 111 patients. *Am. Heart J.* 93, 735 (1977).
29. Rosenblueth, A., Garcia Ramos, J., Studies on flutter and fibrillation. *Am. Heart J.* 33, 677 (1947).

At surgery an end-to-side anastomosis was made over the interruption. The ductus appeared friable and haemorrhagic. The ductus suture ruptured on removal of the ductal clamp resulting in a fatal haemorrhage. During surgery part of the aorta at the entrance site of the ductus arteriosus was removed. On microscopic examination it showed that ductal tissue extended into the aorta, a situation more often encountered in cases with an interruption of the aortic arch. This ductal tissue showed severe damage. There were interruptions of the internal elastic lamina and several lacerations extending into the media, containing thrombotic material which protruded into the lumen. In one tear a polymorphonuclear leucocyte infiltrate was present. The media showed extensive edema resulting in a succulent appearing wall with a sponge-like structure (fig. 6).

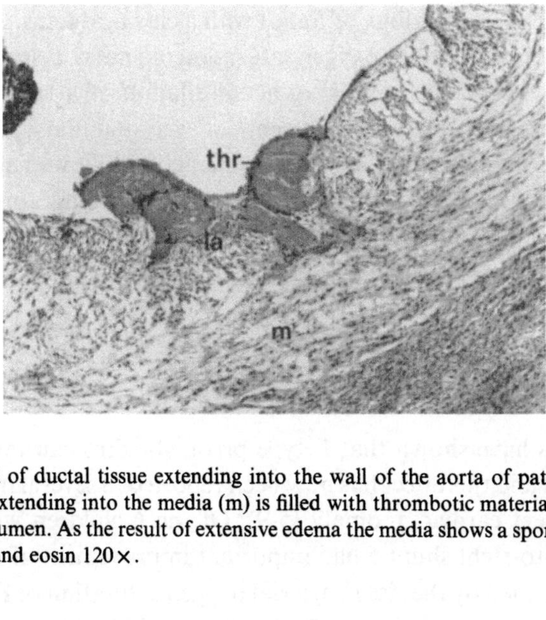

Figure 6. Detail of ductal tissue extending into the wall of the aorta of patient R.L. A large laceration (la) extending into the media (m) is filled with thrombotic material (thr) which protrudes into the lumen. As the result of extensive edema the media shows a sponge-like structure. Haematoxylin and eosin 120×.

N.T. was catheterized at two days of age. A diagnosis of asplenia syndrome was made with pulmonary atresia and persistent ductus, mono-atrium, monoventricle and dextrocardia. After prostaglandin was given the pH improved from 7.29 to 7.34, the PaO_2 rose from 36 to 39 mm Hg and the oxygen concentration from 75 to 81%. No side effects were seen, the PaO_2 stabilized and the patient could be discharged in a reasonable condition.

C.G. was first catheterized at the age of two months. She had a pulmonary atresia with ventricular septal defect and well developed bronchial and intercostal collateral arteries supplying the lung. The ductus was closed at its pulmonary end and this persisted even after performance of the prostaglandin test in the catheterization laboratory.

N.J. was seen for the first time at the age of two months and was markedly cyanotic. At cardiac catheterization a diagnosis of transposition of the great arteries with patent ductus was established. After a balloon septostomy the PaO_2 rose from 20 to 33 m Hg and the oxygen saturation from 66 to 73%. A further increase to 40 mm Hg and 81% followed prostaglandin infusion. On aortography the ductus clearly appeared dilated after the test. Side-effects were not seen and the patient was discharged in a good condition. Four months later the ductus still was widely patent. An arterial switch operation was performed successfully.

E.V. was admitted at about five months of age in a fairly acute cyanotic state. He had a severe tetralogy of Fallot with a closing ductus. After prostaglandin trial the PaO_2 and the oxygen saturation did not rise significantly, but on aortography there was a striking acute dilation of a long meandering ductus and considerable improvement of the pulmonary circulation. Temporary flushing of the left arm and the left chest followed and slight rise of temperature was seen. A shunt between the ascending aorta and right pulmonary artery (Waterston) was carried out on the following day and two weeks later the child was discharged from hospital.

DISCUSSION

In vitro studies have shown that E type prostaglandins can reverse ductus constriction (4) and this effect has now been reported in several infants with a ductus dependent cardiac anomaly (5-9). Of the 6 children with a ductus dependent left-to-right shunt 5 had important improvement of their clinical condition confirmed by the rise in arterial oxygen saturation or PaO_2. In 3 of these an obvious dilatory effect on the ductus could be seen on the angiocardiogram after the prostaglandin E_1 test. The infant of two months of age with a pulmonary atresia and ventricular septal defect totally failed to react to prostaglandin because the ductus had already closed.

The clinical condition of the 2 infants with a ductus dependent right-to-left shunt improved on prostaglandin administration. This was confirmed by normalization of the blood gases. In one of these cases the dilation of the ductus and the increase of the right-to-left shunt was visualized by angiocardiography.

Transient pyrexia occurred on four occasions and an obvious flush reaction was seen in 3 infants over the perfused area but this disappeared when the catheter was removed from the vicinity of the subclavian artery and repositioned in the aortic arch near the ductus. In 1 patient apnoeic spells necessitated assisted ventilation. A state of renal shock was confirmed at post-mortem in one case.

All these side-effects were directly related to the potent action of prostaglandin. The pyrexia and the flush reaction were transient. The apnoeic spells required assisted ventilation. We could not reverse the hypotension and renal shock which appeared after creation of a Waterston in one of our patients.

In three cases the ductus could be measured post-mortem. The measurements were compared with untreated ductus from similar heart malformations (10). The ductus in the prostaglandin treated group tends to be longer and wider indicating that it may be dilated and overstretched. Microscopic examination revealed conspicuous edema of the media of the ductal wall caused by an increased permeability of the vessel wall, this being one of the known side-effects of prostaglandin (12, 13). A similar edema of the vessel wall in systemic arteries is seen during the early phase of malignant hypertension and after experimentally induced hypertension (14, 15). Because of the edema the ductal wall is succulent and friable which may account for the fact that mechanical forces, for instance increased blood flow, have a damaging effect on the ductal wall, causing numerous interruptions of the internal elastic lamina, together with intimal damage and even lacerations extending into the media. The presence of thrombus formation indicates that the damage has not been caused post-mortem. Except in one of our cases, in which problems arose at surgery, with a rupture of the suture and fatal haemorrhage no serious complications as a result of ductal weakening are known.

Despite the recorded side-effects which may occur and the evidence of damaging effects on the ductal wall after prostaglandin E_1 administration, we feel that this new drug has a place in paediatric cardiology, particularly to improve the condition of neonates with ductus dependent cardiac malformations awaiting emergency catheterization and operation.

In view of the observations made on the ductal walls it seems advisable to administer the drug only in a low dose and for a short duration. More needs to be known concerning the possible toxicity of prostaglandin and the effects on other arteries. Additionally more must be known about its toxicity with respect to other therapeutic uses of this drug in man and its possible long-term application (16).

REFERENCES

1. Euler, U. S. Von, Zur Kenntnis der pharmakologischen Wirkungen von Nativsekreten und Extrakten männlicher accessorischer Geschlechtsdrüsen. *Arch. exp. Path. Pharmakol.* 175, 78 (1934).
2. Karim, S. M., *Prostaglandins: physiological, pharmacological and pathological aspects.* Lancaster 1976.
3. Samuelsson, B. and Paoletti, R., *Advances in prostaglandin and thromboxane research.* New York, 1976.
4. Starling, M. B. and Elliott, R. B., The effect of prostaglandins, prostaglandin inhibitors and oxygen on the closure of the ductus arteriosus, pulmonary arteries and umbilical vessels in vitro. *Prostaglandins* 8, 187 (1974).
5. Olley, P. M., Coceani, F. and Bodach, E., E type prostaglandins – a new emergency therapy for certain cyanotic congenital heart malformations. *Circulation* 53, 728 (1976).
6. Radford, D. J., Bloom, K. R., Coceani, D. J., Fariello, R. and Olley, P. M., Prostaglandin E_1 for interrupted aortic arch in neonate. *Lancet* 2, 95 (1976).
7. Rudolph, A. M. and Heymann, M. A., Medical treatment of the ductus arteriosus. *Hospital Practice* 57 (feb. 1977).
8. Neutze, J. M., Starling, M. B., Elliott, R. B. and Barratt-Boyes, M. B., Palliation of cyanotic congenital heart disease in infancy with E-type prostaglandins. *Circulation* 55, 238 (1977).
9. Moulaert, A., Senders, R., van Ertbruggen, I., Huysmans, H. A. and Harinck, E., Effect of E_1 type prostaglandin on hypoxemia in a cyanotic congenital malformation. *Eur. J. Cardiol.* 5, 321 (1977).
10. Gittenberger-De Groot, A. C., Persistent ductus arteriosus: most probably a primary congenital malformation. *Br. Heart J.* 34, 610 (1977).
11. Jatene, A. D., Fontes, V. F., Paulista, P. P., Souza, L. C., Neger, F., Galantier, M. and Sousa, J. E., Anatomic correction of transposition of the great vessels. *J. Thor. Cardiovasc. Surg.* 72, 364 (1976).
12. Solomon, L. M., Juhlin, L., and Kirschenbaum, M. B., Prostaglandin on cutaneous vasculature. *J. Investigative Dermatology* 51, 280 (1968).
13. Persaud. T. V. N., Pregnancy and progeny in rats treated with prostaglandin E_2. *Prostaglandins* 3, 299 (1973).
14. Gardner, D. L., and Matthews, M. A., Ultrastructure of the wall of small arteries in early experimental rat hypertension. *J. Pathology* 97, 51 (1969).
15. Heptinstall, R. H., *Pathology of the Kidney*, 2nd ed., vol. I, p. 142, Boston, 1974.
16. Moulaert, A., Gittenberger, A. and Harinck, E., Prostaglandin and damage to ductus arteriosus. *Lancet* I, 703 (1977).

19. DUCTUS ARTERIOSUS AND INDOMETHACIN

E. HARINCK AND A. J. MOULAERT

INTRODUCTION

Patency of the ductus arteriosus is essential to life in neonates with ductus dependent congenital heart disease such as pulmonary atresia, severe coarctation and interruption of the aorta, but in preterm infants recovering from respiratory distress syndrome it maybe life threatening. The large left-to-right shunt through the ductus may lead to intractable cardiac failure, a complication well-known in neonatal intensive care units. Although medical management is often successful, surgical ligation of the ductus at times is necessary as a life-saving procedure (1-6). In preterm infants, particularly the very small ones, this surgical intervention carries an additional risk. For this reason investigators have searched for less traumatic ways to close the ductus.

From animal experiments it is known that indomethacin constricts the ductus arteriosus by inhibiting the synthesis of the E-type prostaglandins which dilate the ductus (7-12). Elliott and associates reported pharmacological constriction of the ductus in a newborn infant with indomethacin (13). Evidence for constriction of the ductus in preterm infants was reported by Friedman et al. and Heymann et al. (14-16). Constriction of the ductus was nearly always accompanied by disappearance or at least marked reduction of the left-to-right shunt within 24-48 hours of the administration of indomethacin. Transient renal insufficiency was observed to occur in some of the infants as a probable complication of indomethacin treatment. Because of the otherwise encouraging results, however, the authors recommended this pharmacological closure in preference to surgical ligation in these cases. Nadas, commenting on their recommendation, sounded a note of caution (17)! In view of the complications reported to occur in both adults and children with indomethacin treatment he suggested that in general surgical ligation should be preferred to this pharmacological closure until more is known concerning the overall efficacy and toxicity in neonates.

To date we have used this pharmacological approach in 17 preterm infants. In this paper we report our experiences with this drug.

MATERIALS AND METHODS

The infants were admitted to the neonatal intensive care unit of the Wilhelmina Children's Hospital in Utrecht because of hyaline membrane disease or other respiratory problems such as asphyxia and apnoeic spells. The gestational periods varied from 26-33½ weeks and birthweights from 980 to 2020 grams. All infants were critically ill with intractable cardiac failure at the time indomethacin was administered. Before the administration of the drug the infants had a loud systolic or continuous murmur that had not been present on admission, bounding pulses, tachycardia, a heaving cardiac impulse and hepatomegaly. The infants who were on assisted ventilation when they received the drug showed deterioration of their respiratory status, as evidenced by decreasing lung compliance with increasing inspiratory pressures and falling arterial oxygen concentration. The infants still breathing spontaneously had tachypnoea, pulmonary crepitations, hypoxia and respiratory acidosis. The chest X-rays of all infants showed cardiomegaly. Left atrial enlargement was present, as judged by the left atrium to aortic root ratio on the echocardiogram in the 12 cases in whom serial echocardiography was carried out before and after administration of the drug (18, 19).

The indomethacin was administered 6-40 days after birth by nasogastric tube or rectally. The first 6 infants received single doses of 2-3.75 mg/kg on two consecutive days. In the following 11 infants the dose was reduced to 0.1-0.3 mg/kg given once only. In a few cases this dose was repeated within 24 hours because of the inefficacy of the initial dose. A total dose of 0.6 mg/kg was not exceeded.

Improved ventilatory status, obvious softening or disappearance of the precordial murmur, definite radiographic reduction of pulmonary vascular markings and of the size of the heart, decrease of the left atrial/aortic (LA/Ao) root ratio and reduction of hepatomegaly were taken as evidence for constriction of the ductus.

Any untoward effects observed within the first 48 hours of the administration of the drug and which had not been present directly before that time were regarded as possible toxic effects of the drug.

RESULTS

Closure of the ductus or at least marked reduction of the left-to-right shunt occurred in 6 of the 6 infants who had received the large doses within one to two days of the drug administration. This was also observed in 7 of the 11 infants who had received the smaller doses. Of the 4 infants who did not respond in that period of time 2 showed signs of closure three days after the initial treatment. One responded favourably shortly after a second treatment four days later and in another infant signs of closure were observed four days after treatment which probably occurred spontaneously.

Reopening of the ductus with reappearance of the cardiac failure occurred in 5 infants three to seven days after initial constriction. In one infant this occurred on three separate occasions after indomethacin administration. By the third time the left-to-right shunt was smaller than on the previous reopenings and the ductus eventually closed spontaneously. In another infant reopening was observed twice and both times with return of severe cardiac failure which promptly disappeared after surgical ligation of the ductus. These 2 infants had been treated with the smaller doses. In the other three who had received the larger doses the ductus reopened in the presence of increasing pulmonary embarrassment. All three infants died.

Of the three deaths one infant died as result of severe bronchopulmonary dysplasia ten days after the administration of indomethacin, the other two both members of a triplet birth died of bronchopneumonia, seven days after indomethacin was given.

The LA/Ao root ratio's on the echocardiograms before and after the drug administration of the 12 infants in whom serial echocardiography was carried out are shown in fig. 1. In the majority of cases marked reduction of this ratio was observed shortly after the drug administration.

In addition to the beneficial effects of the indomethacin a number of mild to severe clinical problems were observed within 48 hours of its administration (table 1). They were observed in 3 of the 6 infants who had been treated with the larger doses and in 7 of the 11 infants treated with the smaller doses. Some of the infants had more than one complication. Transient renal insufficiency was observed only in the group of infants treated with the larger doses, however, in the infants treated with the smaller doses vomiting, gross abdominal distention with diminished or absent bowel sounds, melaena, necrotising enterocolitis necessitating bowel resection, and exacerbations of lower respiratory tract infections were seen. Some of these were observed with total doses as low as 0.2 and 0.3 mg/kg.

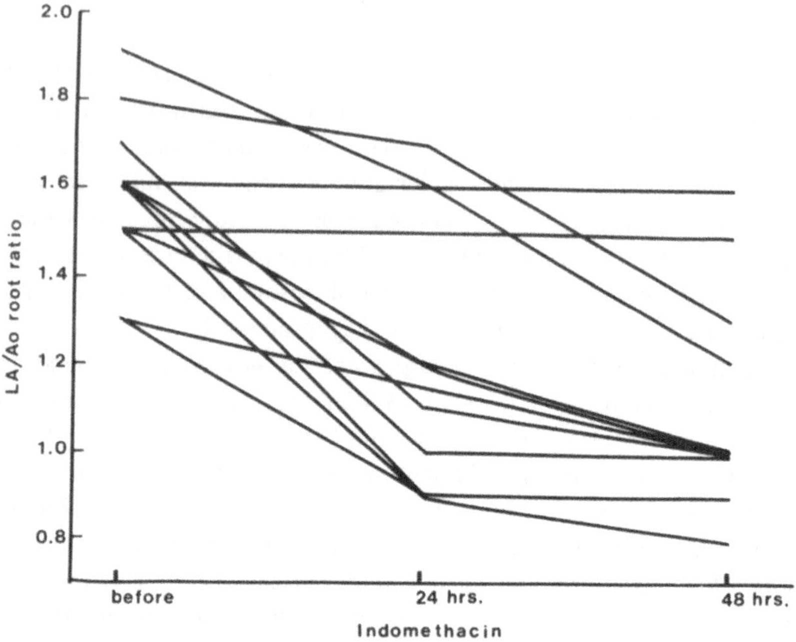

Figure 1. The left atrial/aortic (LA/Ao) root ratio's of 12 preterm infants before and respectively 24 and 48 hours after indomethacin administration.

Table 1. Possible complications of indomethacin.

Type of complication	incidence	
	large dose (n = 3/6)*	low dose (n = 7/11)*
GASTRO-INTESTINAL		
Mild	3	–
Moderate to severe (requiring total parenteral feeding for > 5 days)	–	4
Necrotising enterocolitis	–	1
BRONCHO-PNEUMONIA	–	3
TRANSIENT RENAL FAILURE	2	–

* Number of infants in whom complications occurred and the total number treated with indomethacin.

DISCUSSION

Our results confirm those of Heymann et al., Friedman et al. and Rudolph et al. (14, 15, 16, 20) that in fact indomethacin has a constricting effect on the patent ductus arteriosus in preterm infants and often causes a sudden and dramatic clinical improvement.

Because of our limited experience and because of individual differences in response we have not yet been able to establish the lowest effective dose. Whereas obvious reduction of the left-to-right shunt was observed after a total dose of 0.2 mg/kg a total dose of 0.6 mg/kg could be ineffective.

Although we found no effect with the lowest dose used (0.1 mg/kg), Heymann and associates apparently used this low dose with success (15) and adopted the routine of an initial dose of 0.1 mg/kg, if no effect was observed within 6 hours this same dose was repeated and again 6 hours later if necessary (20). Combining their experiences Friedman, Heymann and Rudolph recommended an initial single oral dose of 0.2 mg/kg to be repeated at 12- to 24-hours intervals if constriction of the ductus has been inadequate. Operative ligation is considered if a total dose of 0.6 mg/kg does not control ductal left-to-right shunting (16). If indomethacin is administered by rectal route good blood levels may be expected and seems to cause less gastrointestinal irritation than the oral route, although local irritation may occur (21).

Delayed closure occurred on a few occasions in the group of infants who had received the smaller doses. This was also observed by Heymann and associates (15).

Normally anatomic closure of the ductus in the neonate may not occur until a few days or even three weeks after physiological closure has occurred (20, 22). Indomethacin causes only physiological closure as result of constriction. Because of this the ductus may reopen later with return of cardiac failure. Apparently this phenomenon is not related to the total dose administered as we observed this after small and large doses.

From our experience with these and other preterm infants with a patent ductus arteriosus we conclude, as have others, that the echocardiogram provides additional valuable information in the management of these neonates (14, 15, 18, 19). Variations of the left-to-right shunt often altered the left atrial/aortic root ratio before they noticeably influenced the cardiac size on the chest X-ray.

We observed transient renal insufficiency as a probable complication of indomethacin in two infants treated with large doses (3.75 mg/kg on two consecutive days). Friedman et al., Heymann et al., also reported transient renal insufficiency in preterm infants after the administration of relatively large doses of indomethacin (14, 15, 16, 20). Unlike previous investigators we observed a number of additional complications. Some of them, as for instance transient renal insufficiency, may have been the result of large doses and, therefore, can be prevented. Nevertheless, it should be noted that they may occur also after the administration of small doses. Obviously any or all complications we observed may be consequence of the disease process itself in these small and critically ill neonates. However, their occurrence so soon after the drug administration should at least serve as a warning that complications may occur even when total doses as low as 0.2-0.3 mg/kg are used, particularly since side-effects are well known to occur in older children and adults, even during brief trials (21, 23, 24).

Despite possible toxic effects of indomethacin we feel that with the proper available facilities there is a place for the indomethacin in the treatment of preterm infants suffering from intractable cardiac failure who otherwise would have to undergo ligation of the ductus. However, only very small doses should be used and the infant should not suffer any complication known to be a suspect side-effect of the drug.

REFERENCES

1. Siassi, B., Emmanouilides, G. C., Cleveland, R. J. and Hirose, F., Patent ductus arteriosus complicating prolonged assisted ventilation in respiratory distress syndrome. *J. Pediat.* 74, 11 (1969).
2. Kitterman, J. A., Edmunds, L. H., Jr., Gregory, G. A., Heymann, M. A., Tooley, W. H. and Rudolph, A. M., Patent ductus arteriosus in premature infants. *New Engl. J. Med.* 287, 474 (1972).
3. Zachman, R. D., Ledbetter, M. K., Botham, R. J., Steinmetz, G. P. and Graven, S. N., Incidence and treatment of patent ductus arteriosus in the low weight neonate. *Pediat. Res.* 6, 81 (1972).
4. Gupta, J. M., Van Vliet, P. K. J., Fisk, G. C. and Wright, J. S., Ductus ligation in respiratory distress syndrome. *J. Thorac. Cardiovasc. Surg.* 63, 642 (1972).
5. Zachman, R. D., Steinmetz, G. P., Botham, R. J., Graven, S. N., Ledbetter, M. K., Incidence and treatment of the patent ductus arteriosus in the ill premature neonate. *Am. Heart J.* 87, 697 (1974).
6. Lees, M. H,, Commentary: Patent ductus arteriosus in premature infants – A diagnostic procedure. *J. Pediat.* 86, 132 (1975).
7. Starling, M. B. and Elliott, R. B., The effect of prostaglandins, prostaglandin inhibitors and oxygen on the closure of the ductus arteriosus, pulmonary arteries and umbilical vessels in vitro. *Prostaglandins* 8, 187 (1974).
8. Sharpe, G. L., Thalme, B. and Larsson, K. S., Studies on closure of ductus arteriosus XI. Ductal closure in utero by a prostaglandin synthesis inhibitor. *Prostaglandins* 8, 363 (1974).

9. Coceani, F., Olley, P. M. and Bodach, E., Lamb ductus arteriosus: Effect of prostaglandin synthesis inhibitors on the muscle tone and the response to prostaglandin-E. *Prostaglandins* 9, 292 (1975).
10. Sharpe, G. L., Larsson, K. S. and Thalme, B., Studies on closure of the ductus arteriosus XII. In utero effect of indomethacin and sodium salicylate in rats and rabbits. *Prostaglandins* 9, 585 (1975).
11. Sharpe, G. L., Thalme, B. and Larsson, K. S., Ductal closure in utero by a prostaglandin synthetase inhibitor. *Pediat. Res.* 9, 271 (1975).
12. Coceani, F., Olley, P. M., Bishai, I., Bodach, E., Heaton, J., Nashat, M. and White, E., Prostaglandins and the control of muscle tone in the ductus arteriosus. In: Reivick (ed.), *Advances in experimental medicine and biology*. Plenum, New York (in press).
13. Elliott, R. B., Starling, M. B. and Neutze, J. M., Medical manipulation of the ductus arteriosus. *Lancet* 1, 140 (1975).
14. Friedman, W. F., Hirschklau, M. J., Morton, P. P., Pitlick, P. T. and Kirkpatrick, S. E., Pharmacological closure of patent ductus arteriosus in the premature infant. *New Engl. J. Med.* 295, 526 (1976).
15. Heymann, M. A., Rudolph, A. M. and Silverman, N. H., Closure of the ductus arteriosus in premature infants by inhibition of prostaglandin synthesis. *New Engl. J. Med.* 295, 530 (1976).
16. Friedman, W. F., Heymann, M. A., Rudolph, A. M., Commentary: New thoughts on an old problem – Patent ductus arteriosus in the premature infant. *J. Pediat.* 90, 338 (1977).
17. Nadas, A. S., Patent ductus revised. *New Engl. J. Med.* 295, 563 (1976).
18. Silverman, N. H., Lewis, A. B., Heymann, M. A. and Rudolph, A. M., Echocardiographic assessment of ductus arteriosus shunts in premature infants. *Circulation* 50, 821 (1974).
19. Baylen, B. G., Meyer, R. A., Kaplan, S., Ringenburg, W. E. and Korfhagen, U. T., Critically ill premature infant with patent ductus arteriosus and pulmonary disease. An echocardiographic assessment. *J. Pediat.* 86, 423 (1975).
20. Rudolph, A. M. and Heymann, M. A., Medical treatment of the ductus arteriosus. *Hospital Practice* 12, 57 (1977).
21. O'Brien, W. M., Indomethacin: A survey of clinical trials. *Clin. Pharmacol. Ther.* 9, 94 (1968).
22. Rudolph, A. M., Closure of the ductus arteriosus. In: Rudolph, A. M. (ed.), *Congenital diseases of the heart*. Chicago 1974.
23. Martindale. Indomethacin. *The Extra Pharmacopoeia*. A. Wade (ed.), 26th ed., 237 (1973).
24. Solomon, L., Activation of latent infection by indomethacin: A report of three cases. *Br. Med. J.* 1, 961 (1966).

20. FLOW AND PRESSURE: THE MECHANICS OF CLOSURE OF THE HUMAN DUCTUS ARTERIOSUS

C. L. D. C. BRUINS AND A. C. GITTENBERGER-DE GROOT

MORPHOLOGY

In physiology there is a reciprocal influence between form and function. The relative size of blood vessels immediately after birth gives us some information on flow distribution before birth. On post mortem examination this is valid for elastic vessels like aorta and pulmonary artery, but less so for muscular vessels like the ductus arteriosus, where the size mainly depends on the amount of muscular contraction.

Ductal size was measured in human specimens of different antenatal length and postnatal age (1). Comparison of the data (fig. 1) suggests the following changes. The cross-sectional area of the ductus lumen remains unchanged while the ductus wall shows increasing thickness in the last foetal months. During or immediately after birth the ductus is widely patent. Functional closure by muscular contraction occurs gradually during the first day.

These conclusions are in agreement with the following physiological data. Aortic and pulmonary arterial pressure are no longer necessarily equal before birth, the aortic pressure usually being somewhat lower. Just after birth a reversal of flow through the ductus takes place and twelve hours later the ductus is functionally closed. As postmortem manipulation of the ductus causes it to contract, the findings of Odé (1) could be based on an artefact, the amount of muscular tissue and thus of contraction increasing with foetal age. However, this would not explain the wide ductus, found in cases of death shortly after full term delivery. Hörnblad (3) found, on total body freezing with fixation of neonates and near-term foetuses of mice, rats and pigs a patent ductus at birth. Functional closure took 10 minutes to 2 hours. Only the rabbit and the guinea pig showed an increase in wall thickness at, but not before birth. Changes in wall structure only occurred after birth. His method prevents contraction by manipulation. He sees the closure as a solitary occurrence, intended as conclusive. It is still very questionable if this is also valid for human beings.

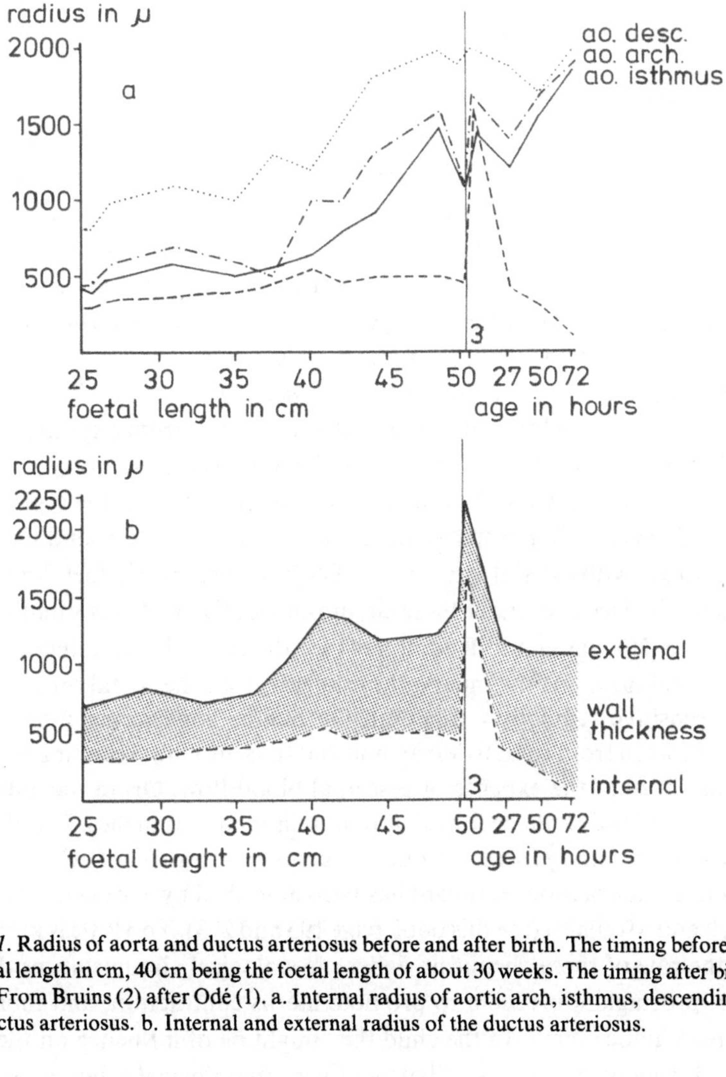

Figure 1. Radius of aorta and ductus arteriosus before and after birth. The timing before birth is by foetal length in cm, 40 cm being the foetal length of about 30 weeks. The timing after birth is in hours. From Bruins (2) after Odé (1). a. Internal radius of aortic arch, isthmus, descending aorta and ductus arteriosus. b. Internal and external radius of the ductus arteriosus.

CIRCUMSTANCES INFLUENCING CLOSURE

Functional closure of the ductus is effected by muscular contraction. In human neonates it is less sudden than in some mammals (4). It is reversible during the first days, as long as no anatomical sealing has started. Physiological causes for reopening are all circumstances that lead to increasing pulmonary pressure, such as bowel movement or crying. The effect of contraction depends on the stimulation, on eventual counterforces, and on the structure of the ductus wall.

1. Stimulation to contraction

It is well known that *oxygen tension* of blood in the ductus and in its adventitial and medial vessels (vasa vasorum) plays an important role. The sensitivity to oxygen increases with foetal age, in lambs this occurs in the last of the five months of gestation. The normal rise after birth in oxygen tension from below 25 to above 50 mmHg is sufficient to stimulate the musculature to forceful contraction. In terms of oxygen saturation of foetal haemoglobin this corresponds to a rise from 55% or less to at least 90%.

The ductus has a *vagal* as well as a *sympathetic innervation.* The adrenergic system seems to be of little influence on ductus closure from oxygen rise after birth, but the release of acetylcholine, on the other hand, may play a positive role. It is unknown what the function is of the extensive adrenergic innervation which is rich in norepinephrine. In extremely hypoxic conditions like foetal distress, with arterial saturations of 40% or less, a rise in foetal catecholamines takes place and under these circumstances the ductus is stimulated to contraction. Heymann and Rudolph (4) see the relaxed foetal ductus as the normal condition, but the innervation suggests that the foetal ductus could have a sensitive regulatory function. On ductus contraction more blood would be forced from right to left atrium and thus into the ascending aorta, to heart and head at the expense of placental blood flow. Or, in the antenatal phase, more blood could be forced into the pulmonary branches. The effect of an infusion of some *prostaglandins* as ductus relaxans or of *prostaglandin inhibitors* as contraction stimulant has been described by Moulaert et al. and Harinck and Moulaert (see this book page 193 and 203). Too little is known as yet of the role of these chemicals under physiological circumstances. In the mother, prostaglandins seem to promote uterus contraction, and thus they might help induce birth. In the child they might be of influence on the neonatal widening of the ductus. Whatever their physiological function may be, they are short-lived and easily broken down. Other *chemicals* like bradykinin may have some influence.

2. The effect of ductus contraction

The effect depends partly on the counterforce of the *lateral pressure* inside the ductus.

This is determined in more than one way by the size of the ductus, and by the aortic and pulmonary artery pressure. Once the ductus begins to narrow,

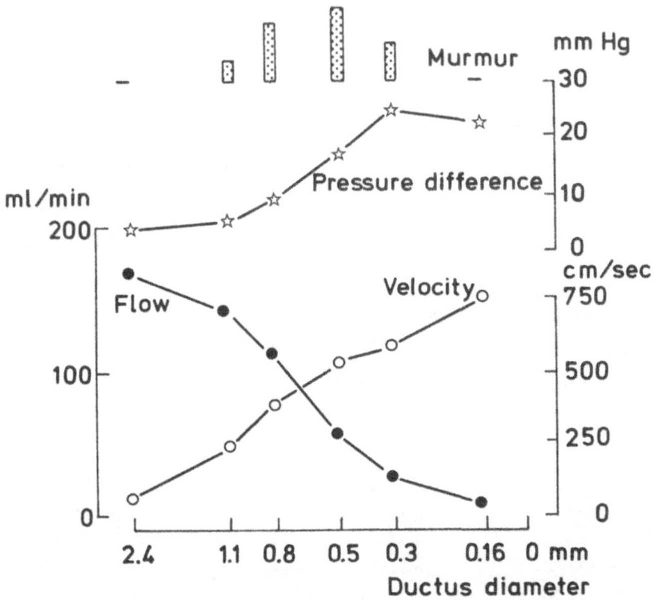

Figure 2. A composition of changes in murmur, aortopulmonary pressure difference, ductus flow and its linear velocity with decreasing ductus size in lamb with open chest under positive pressure ventilation. After Dawes (8).

the ductal flow can no longer prevent an increasing pressure gradient between aorta and pulmonary artery (see later). A systolic pressure difference of up to 40 mmHg may be established in a short vessel of about 5 mm length. The ductus resistance must by that time be high. Figure 2 shows what can be interpreted as the effect of progressive narrowing of the ductus. The ductus flow decreases although an increasing pressure gradient develops, causing an increasing velocity of blood through the ductus. This causes turbulence in the pulmonary artery producing vibration of its wall, which gives rise to a murmur. Beyond a certain degree of narrowing, flow and murmur decrease even if pressure gradient and velocity still increase. The data are from Dawes et al. (5), measured in mature foetal lambs.

According to Bernoulli's principle of constant total energy, increase in kinetic energy, that is in speed, is compensated by a loss in potential energy, as lateral pressure. The lateral pressure in the ductus at its pulmonary end thus could well be, on theoretical basis, 10 mmHg or more below the pulmonary artery pressure. The ductus contents in that region would offer no opposition to its functional closure, on the contrary, a Venturi effect might be present, with alternating flow acceleration and ductus closure. Closure in a ductus normally starts at the pulmonary side.

3. The structure of the ductal wall

The wall of the ductus consists of an intima, an elastic layer, the thick muscular media and an adventitia. In a neonate of at least 35 weeks gestation normally the histological changes conducive to closure are present: cushions of intimal tissue, fragmentation of the internal elastic lamina, changes in the internal muscular layer (fig. 3a). These intimal cushions have little influence on flow in a distended ductus, but once the ductus starts contracting they form an extra resistance to flow. It is because of them that functional closure is so effective. After functional closure the remnants of the lumen are gra-

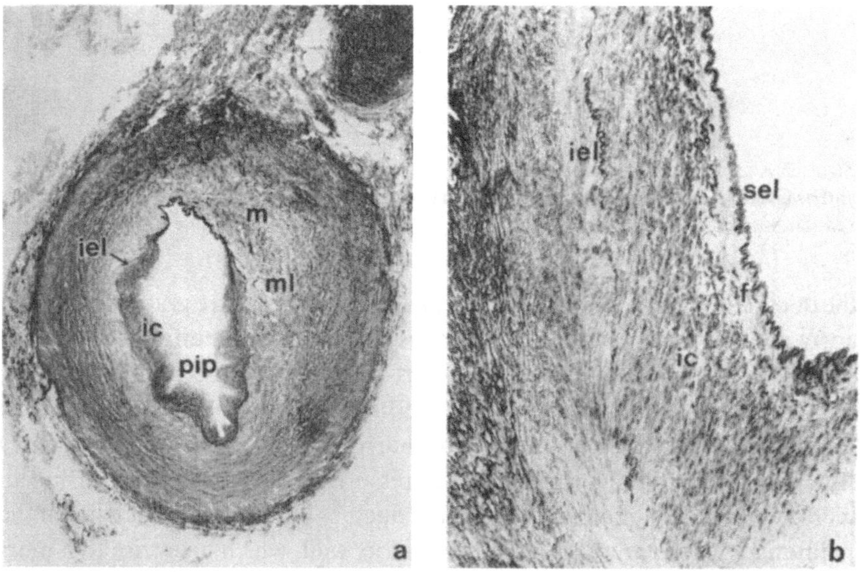

Figure 3a. Cross-section of the ductus arteriosus of a 12 days old premature, gestational age 36 weeks. Intimal cushions (ic) protrude into the lumen showing all features essential for a normal anatomical closing process. Underneath the cushions the internal elastic lamina (iel) is fragmented while on top of the intimal cushions there is already some postnatal intima proliferation (pip) with complete lack of elastic fibres. Also in the media (m) mucoid lakes (ml) are present. Van Gieson elastic tissue stain, 22 ×.

Figure 3b. Part of the wall of a persistent ductus arteriosus of a 7 months old infant. Underneath the intimal cushions (ic) there is a fragmented internal elastic lamina (iel) and additionally bordering the lumen there is a thick subendothelial elastic lamina (sel) which is seen very often in case of persistent ductus arteriosus. Van Gieson elastic tissue stain, 43 ×.

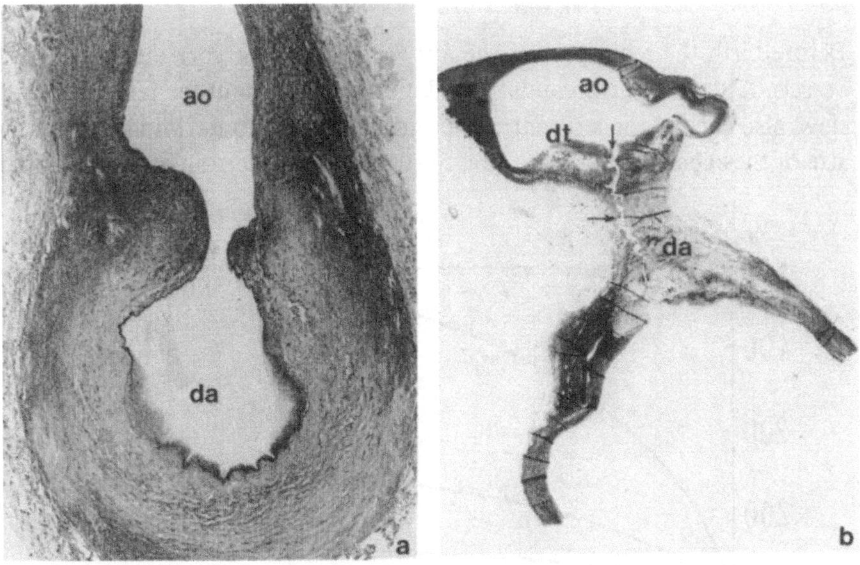

Figure 4. Longitudinal sections of the area where the ductus enters the aorta. a. The same case as pictured in fig. 3a. The ductus arteriosus (da) differs markedly from the aorta (ao) in containing much less elastic material. Van Gieson elastic tissue stain, 22 ×. b. Ductus of a 3 weeks old infant with a coarctation and a ventricular septal defect. The ductus arteriosus (da) was very wide and is now almost closed (arrows: artificial lumen). Abundant ductal tissue (dt) protrudes into the lumen of the aorta (ao). Van Gieson elastic tissue stain, 5 ×.

dually filled by secondary intimal fibrous proliferation. Normally the elastic lamellae of the aorta merge for the greater part into the adventitia, a smaller part forming the internal elastic lamina (fig. 4a). In cases with VSD where there is a large ductus and a smaller isthmus we can demonstrate that the abundant ductus wall tissue partly protrudes into the descending aorta (fig. 4a, b). This might be the result of neonatal contraction. The mechanism in temporary coarctation, loss of pulse pressure in caudal arteries with cranial hypertension, described in infants after surgical, and in rare cases after spontaneous ductus closure (6) is probably identical. Surgical ductus closure and probably forceful neonatal contraction as well, are a traumatic event, causing temporary oedema of the ductal wall.

PHYSIOLOGY

Before birth the main part of the *left ventricular flow* goes into the cranial vessels. After birth, the caudal circulation, be it without the large placental flow, also depends on left ventricular output. The postnatal initial decrease in size of the superior vena cava (fig. 5) suggests that the cranial flow becomes

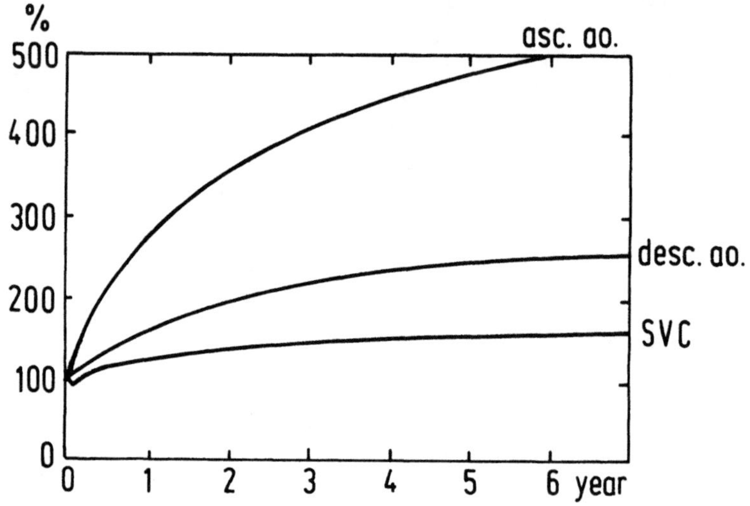

Figure 5. Increase in internal circumference of ascending and descending aorta and superior vena cava with age. The point of reference is 100% at birth. From Handbook of circulation (7).

smaller in this phase. The narrow praeductal aorta, the isthmus, is stretched open, its flow is increased to at least twice the antenatal value, which is enough to provide an aorto-pulmonary shunt through the ductus as well. Still, the isthmus may be recognizable by its smaller size during the first year of life. In agreement with this is the fact that during at least nine months the systolic pressure in the femoral artery is slightly below or equal to the brachial systolic pressure while after that period it becomes 10-15 mmHg higher. Before birth the *right ventricular flow* in mammals is nearly twice the left ventricular flow. It passes mainly through the ductus. After a normal delivery, during which the lungs are compressed and emptied of alveolar fluid, the alveoles, and with them the surrounding capillaries distend with the first inspiration. From that moment pulmonary vascular resistance decreases in the human neonate, so much so that even with a relatively enormous, probably more than threefold

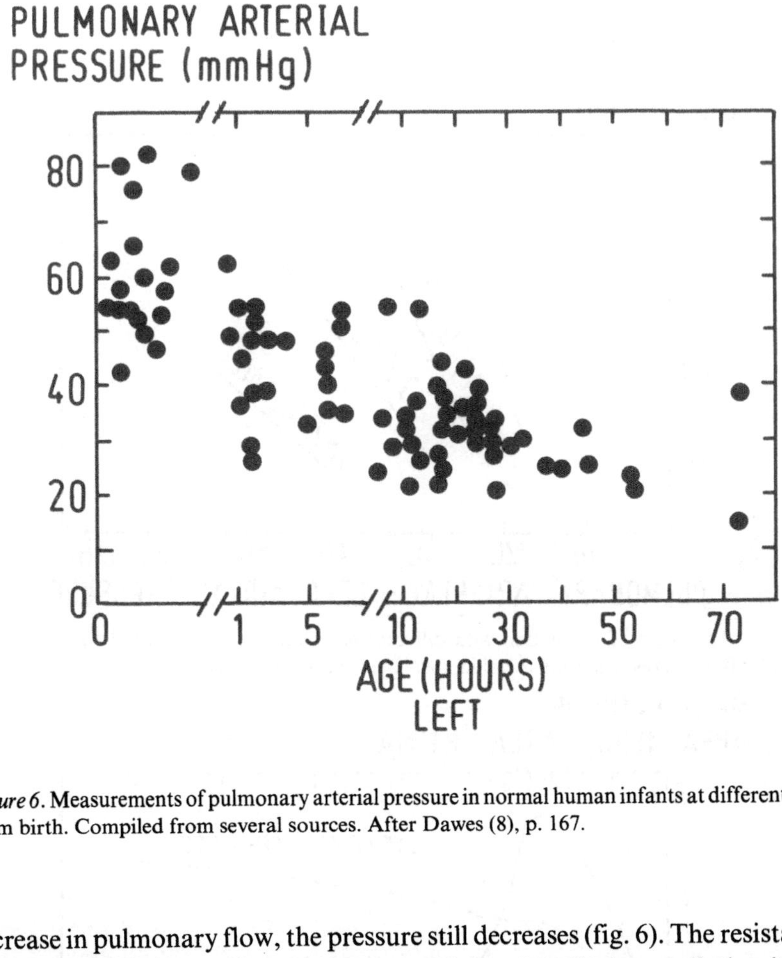

Figure 6. Measurements of pulmonary arterial pressure in normal human infants at different ages from birth. Compiled from several sources. After Dawes (8), p. 167.

increase in pulmonary flow, the pressure still decreases (fig. 6). The resistance lowering influence on the pulmonary vessels is primarily by ventilation itself, but the composition of the gas mixture is also of great importance (8). Room air, relatively rich in oxygen and poor in carbon dioxyde, has a beneficial effect as demonstrated in lambs (fig. 7). After expansion of the capillaries the small, muscular resistance arteries also widen and show a loss of muscular media tissue, Naeye (9) compared the muscular thickness to the thickness of intimal tissue inclusive the internal elastic membrane. Within four weeks the relation is halved (fig. 8). The load on the right ventricle finds its expression in its weight and wall volume, as well as in right preponderance on the electrocardiogram. An antenatal elective increase in right ventricular wall could well be due to antenatal increase in ductus resistance, increase in pressure and pulmonary circulation. After birth the right ventricular pressure decreases,

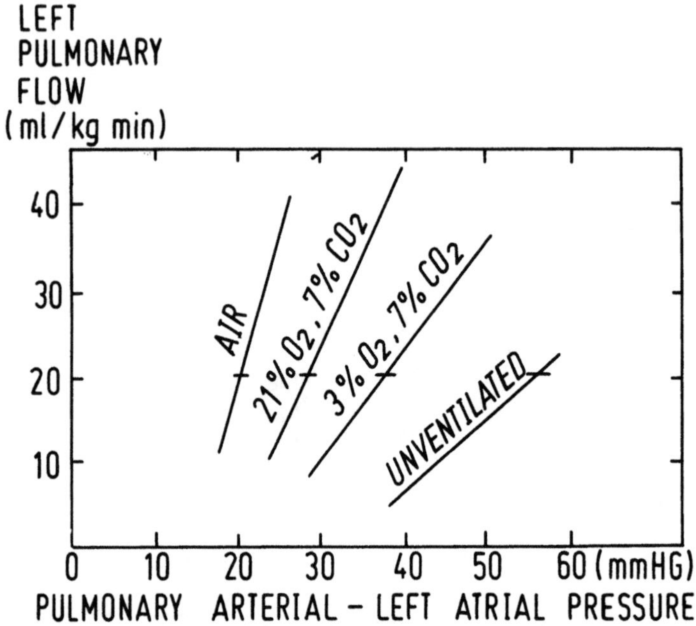

Figure 7. The effect of ventilation with different gas mixtures upon the pulmonary arterial pressure: flow curves in mature foetal lambs. After Dawes (8), p. 84.

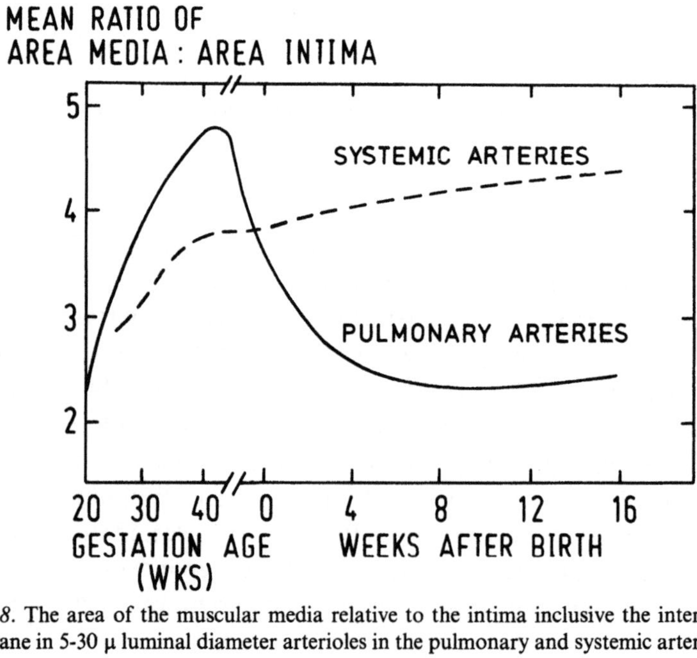

Figure 8. The area of the muscular media relative to the intima inclusive the internal elastic membrane in 5-30 μ luminal diameter arterioles in the pulmonary and systemic arterial beds at different ages from human autopsies. After Naeye (9).

there is a concomitant loss of wall volume. From then on, the left ventricular wall shows an increasing preponderance, as well in wall volume (fig. 9) as, more gradually, on the electrocardiogram.

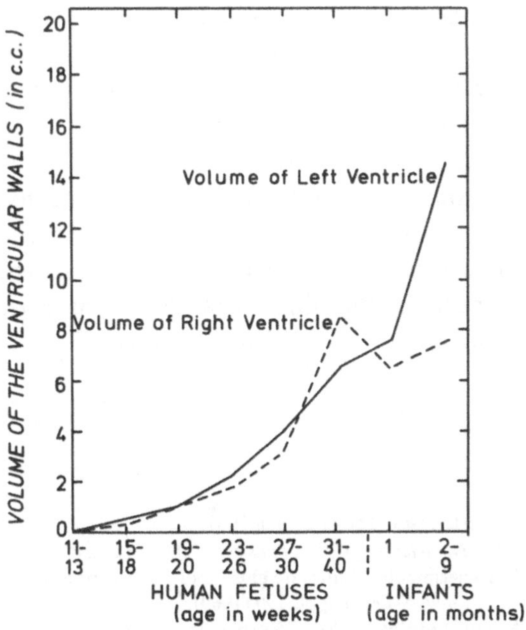

Figure 9. The ratio of muscular volume of right and left ventricular wall in human foetus and infants. From Cassels (10), p. 126. After Sciacca.

After the first day of life the flow through both ventricles is equal. The aorta shows an excessive growth rate during the first months (7), indicating a large increase in left ventricular output (fig. 5). The growth rate of the pulmonary artery, though not included in the figure, is at least equal to that of the aorta.

PATHOLOGY

Delayed ductal closure or *prolonged patency* is a condition of a normal ductus under abnormal haemodynamic circumstances. Even then anatomic sealing is as a rule complete within three months after birth. Prematures, small-for-dates and infants born by caesarean section have more fluid in their lungs (alveoli, interstitium and lymphatic vessels) than mature babies after a normal birth. A neonatal distress syndrome or even hyaline membrane disease may be the result. This leads to a low APGAR score, prolonged high pulmonary vascular resistance and arterial pressure. The result is a very inefficient ductus contraction against a high internal pressure. Neonatal distress after meconium aspiration or any other pulmonary or cerebral affection that causes hypoventilation may initiate a comparable course of events.

Non-closure or *persistent patency* of the ductus is a congenital defect in itself, that may occur either as a single anomaly or as part of a syndrome.

Brundin (11) has shown with a fluorescence technique that in a persistent ductus adrenergic nerves in the muscular media are absent. According to Gittenberger (12) a constant finding in these cases was a subendothelial elastic lamina bordering the lumen (fig. 3b) either as the internal elastic lamina, or as an additional lamina on top of the intimal cushions.

REFERENCES

1. Odé, E., *De ductus arteriosus*. Thesis Leiden 1951.
2. Bruins, C. L. D. C., *De arteriële pool van het hart*. Thesis Leiden 1973.
3. Hörnblad, P. Y., Experimental studies on closure of the ductus arteriosus utilizing whole-body freezing. *Acta Paed. Scand.* suppl. 190 (1969).
4. Heymann, M. A. and Rudolph, A. M., Control of the ductus arteriosus. *Physiol. Review* 55, 62 (1975).
5. Dawes, G. S., Mott, J. C. and Widdicombe, J. G., The cardiac murmur from the patent ductus arteriosus in newborn lambs. *J. Physiol.* 128, 344 (1955).
6. Elseed, A. M., Shinebourne, E. A. and Paneth, M., Manifestation of juxtaductal coarctation after surgical ligation of persistent ductus arteriosus in infancy. *Br. Heart J.* 36, 687 (1974).
7. Scammon, R. A., Studies on the growth and structure of the infant thorax. 1927. Cited in: Dittmar, D. S., et al. (ed.), *Handbook of circulation*. Philadelphia 1959.
8. Dawes, G. S., *Foetal and neonatal physiology*. Chicago 1968.
9. Naeye, R. L., Arterial changes during the perinatal period. *Arch. Pathol.* 71, 121 (1961).
10. Cassels, D. E., *The ductus arteriosus*. Springfield 1973.
11. Brundin, T., Norberg, K. A. and Söderlund, S., Lack of adrenergic nerves in the circular smooth muscles of ductus arteriosus persistens. *Scand. J. Thorac. Cardiovasc. Surg.* 5, 16 (1971).
12. Gittenberger-de Groot, A. C., Persistent ductus arteriosus: most probably a primary congenital malformation. *Br. Heart J.* 39, 610 (1977).

INDEX